Praise for *My Guru Cancer*

"As a cancer nurse for over 30 years who has witnessed the stress and suffering of many people going through cancer, I have never read a book like Bethany Webb's *My Guru Cancer*. She has sensitively and with great integrity and candor shared a new and inspirational way to face and live with cancer, one where peace, humor and love co-exist. She doesn't sugar coat. Her fear and pain are very real. However, through her living example she is offering a roadmap that anyone with an open mind can follow to find true, personal treasure amid the complexities of life with cancer. I highly recommend this book to anyone interested in reframing life's challenges into opportunities for transformation."

—Meg Maley
BSN, RN, Co-founder/CEO of CanSurround

"A moving memoir that showcases the transformative healing that mindfulness and community can bring to one's cancer journey. By reclaiming cancer as a gift, Bethany sheds light on the challenges of a cancer diagnosis as a young adult, while simultaneously opening herself up to healing, community, adventure, and unbridled freedom and peace. She reminds us to look at cancer through a new lens—one of acceptance and opportunity, rather than fear or isolation."

—Brad Ludden
Founder of First Descents

D1452097

"An uplifting, funny, intelligent and powerful story about Bethany's journey with breast cancer. Using The Work of Byron Katie, Bethany took every obstacle and turned them into precious gifts to expand her soul. I personally find her book extremely helpful as I'm also dealing with a serious breast cancer diagnosis. She taught me that it's possible to find levity, laughter and beauty, while facing my own mortality. This book offers a unique perspective to transform shadows into light. I highly recommend it!"

—Tara Coyote
Stage IV Cancer Thriver, Author, Founder of Cancer Warrioress

"What I love most about Bethany Webb's *My Guru Cancer* is the amazingly authentic narrative. It's raw, it's honest, and it has impact. I'm sure it will serve and give heart to many seeking the same true freedom that Bethany found. There is something to be valued in the embrace of what is real and seeing it for what it is, rather than the enemy. It takes courage and this story is packed with courage. It's also a story that is told with love. It's a story of transformation and the power we hold within us to transform, even in a time when most of us would rather not drop the fight as Bethany did and so beautifully articulates. I highly recommend this book to all, with or without a diagnosis, as I believe, the essence of the story is truly an inspiration for all of us."

—Michael Lee
Author, Founder of Phoenix Rising Yoga Therapy

My Guru
CANCER

YOU DON'T HAVE TO FIGHT TO FIND
TRUE FREEDOM FROM THE C WORD

BETHANY WEBB

My Guru Cancer: You Don't Have to Fight to Find True Freedom from the C Word
Published by Mariposa Press
Lakewood, CO

Names: Webb, Bethany, author.
Title: My guru cancer : you don't have to fight to find true freedom from the c word / by Bethany Webb.
Description: First trade paperback original edition. | Lakewood [Colorado] : Mariposa Press, 2020. | Appendices included. | Also published as an ebook.
Identifiers: ISBN 978-1-7352977-0-5
Subjects: LCSH: Breast cancer—Patients—Biography.
BISAC: HEALTH & FITNESS / Women's Health.
Classification: LCC CT275 | DDC 920.9 WEBB–dc22

ISBN: 978-1-7352977-0-5
HEALTH & FITNESS / Women's Health.

Original cover painting by Bethany Webb
Cover and interior design by Victoria Wolf, Wolf Design & Marketing
Wedding photos by Margie Woods, Steph Grant, Leigh Mergehenn Petr
First Descents photos by Melissa Markle

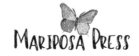

MARIPOSA PRESS

To everyone whose life has been touched by cancer…

It sure is a wild ride

With so much beauty deep inside

Break free from the BS in that sweet mind

And only gratitude and giggles will be left behind

This is for *you.*

xoxo,

Bethany

Contents

1

Life Happens for Me

2:00 AM, AND MY MIND was fully awake. Words were filling my head like a Scrabble tsunami, and all I could hear was: *WRITE. Dictate this mental activity.* I didn't ask questions; I just knew that was what I was supposed to do. *Alrighty.*

Silently, I slipped out of bed without waking my sleeping husband and tiptoed into the living room. The quiet stillness of the corner of our L-shaped mid-century couch invited me: "Empty your brain here, Bethany." *Ummm…do couches talk? Am I losing it?*

Cozy on the sofa with a fuzzy, grey blanket softly wrapped around my shoulders, letters of relief began to pour out onto my bright laptop screen. It felt so good to release my mind onto the glowing digital page. I had no clue if anyone would ever read a word, but that had nothing to do with me.

My job? Listen. Write.

OK, OK…stop yelling at me! Here we go.

1

Over the past few weeks, I had experienced a monumental shift in awareness. Cancer might actually be growing in my 33-year-old, healthy, strong, yoga-practicing, organic-eating body. And the weirdest part? I was totally at peace with it. I went from complete terror to peace. Dare I say—I was even excited! *Ummm… who does that? What the hell is happening here?*

A little less than a year ago, in November, I found a lump in my left breast. It was the size of a pea and moved around like a smooth marble. This one didn't frighten or shock me. My boobs had basically become a rockin' lump factory in my late twenties, so I was quite familiar with the find-a-lump-don't-freak-out-it's-probably-nothing dance routine.

I always took my lumps straight to the doctors, and through manual exams and ultrasounds, every time they had determined they were just cysts or swollen lymph nodes. Because I didn't have health insurance, Planned Parenthood was my go-to place for lady stuff. Health insurance was insanely expensive for self-employed yoga therapists, and it wasn't like I was going to use medicine to heal me anyway if I ever encountered a big issue…I was a natural kind of girl. An "identity" that would soon be put to the ultimate test and blown to smithereens.

I had been told that I had dense breast tissue, and the doctors even had a fancy, sexy name for it: fibrocystic breast disease. This is totally normal, especially for young women. I learned how to monitor the lumps, stay calm, and watch them disappear over time.

Ironically, the November lump was the *only* lump I didn't take to the pros right away. *Ohhh…it's just another cyst. I mean…me? Cancer? I'm one of the healthiest people I know. Not possible. Let's just pour some essential oils on it and send some healing vibes.*

Oh, how I wish I could've tapped my clueless November self on the shoulder and offered a sweet whisper, saying, "Hey dumbass…you don't know shit and are pouring essential oils over tumors…cancer likes to thrive in *any* body, including young, healthy ones! And if you catch it early, treatment plans can be shorter, easier, and decrease your chances of that thing called DEATH." *Sigh.*

But that wasn't my path. And honestly, I don't beat myself up about it. What's the point? What's done is done. I was simply believing my thoughts and too busy living in the prime of my life.

My world in the summer of 2015 was pretty dang awesome. I was in the midst of so many exciting transitions. My husband, Travis, and I had been on-site managers of a bed & breakfast retreat property in the Hill Country near Austin, Texas.

We had gotten married there over four years earlier and had completely fallen in love with the place. I remember when we first toured the property as a wedding venue. We pulled up to the driveway to the sight of a tall adobe straw bale home peeking over the carport. An open doorway framed our first glimpse of the property: magenta and lilac azaleas, towering forest green cedar trees, and a small pond with a stone-white angel fountain. A rustic coyote fence surrounded the other accommodations: a pink cottage and three funky red, blue, and green eco-friendly tiny homes.

"Page? Page Parkes…is that you?" Travis said in complete shock as a stunning, blond-haired woman walked around the corner to greet us. I had been the one in contact with her, as Page and her husband owned the property. Much to my surprise, she was also Travis's previous agent. He had worked for her ten years prior as a model through her modeling agency. (Yes, my hubby used to be a model—something he rarely admits yet I brag about quite often!). The synchronicity of already knowing each other gave me goosebumps.

The owners were living in Houston, and they had purchased the property with the intention of moving there when it came time to retire. Currently, their time was filled to the brim with running their own businesses and raising three young children, so they rented out the property a few times a month in the meantime. They named it Living Waters on Lake Travis. The original owner and builder was an artist, and during the construction of the main house, she buried a vial of holy water underneath a jade gem embedded into the stone flooring. The house is literally built on holy water, hence the name Living Waters. I wasn't super into the whole crystals and prayer beads thing—although maybe I was supposed to be because I was a yogini? Even so, I had to admit that I felt totally mushy and at peace in holy water land.

We took one step into this magical space and immediately knew—we were getting married here. It offered everything we'd ever imagined for our intimate wedding retreat. A large, beautiful home set atop a cliff overlooking the lake, a place where we could all hang out and eat organic, vegetarian meals prepared by our chef. Plenty of accommodations for our close friends and family to stay on-site with us.

An outdoor, open-air pavilion for yoga classes in the mornings and dancing at night. A long, winding stone path, leading to a crushed granite ceremony space by the lake. *Oh wait—what's that sound?* Just the newly installed waterfall cascading down the hill, creating a small pond where we would say, "I do." (I have a seriously special connection with water. Maybe it's because I grew up near the Gulf of Mexico in Ft. Myers, Florida.)

The property was perfect. And so was our wedding retreat. It was, without a doubt, the best weekend of my life. Standing barefoot in my white bohemian wedding dress, a freshly drawn henna tattoo wrapped around my ankle, I looked into Travis's sparkling green eyes. He wore a white, button-down shirt with white linen pants that barely hung over his hips. *Jesus Christ, I can't believe that I get to be with this gorgeous man for the rest of my life. My love, my best friend.* His long brown hair partially covered his right eye as he read his poetic vows to me.

"You've opened my eyes to the reality and wonder of true love. You've shown my heart how to open more than I ever thought possible. I will hold your hand as we walk in love's freedom. I will let go with you in moments of uncontrollable laughter and silliness as we marvel at this life together. I will breathe with you in moments of challenge and growth, assuring you that everything is OK. I will support you as you realize your dreams and express your heart's desire. I will love you always and forever. Thank you for loving me. Thank you for your playful and amazing sense of humor. Thank you for your infinite patience and unwavering support of my dreams and ambitions. Thank you for being in that book store on May 1st."

How incredible is this guy? Butterflies filled the air as I sprung to my tippy-toes, wrapped my arms around his neck, and reached up for our first married kiss. His hands swept around my waist to pull me in closer. It was one of those romantic, sexy wedding kisses that lasts almost a little too long. My heart nearly exploded with happy dance joy. *Could life get any better than this?*

After all of our guests departed...and after some majorly hot sex on the deck of the lookout tower of the straw bale home, my husband and I snuggled up on a wooden bench overlooking the lake. The sun was setting over the Hill Country horizon, creating swirls of orange and yellow glitter on the water's surface. We were overcome by a distinct feeling. The property felt so familiar, so right. We just knew we were meant to do something there, but we didn't know what, when, or how.

It turned out we didn't need to know. Life figured that out for us instead.

A few months after our wedding retreat, out of the blue, our landlord in Dallas informed us that she had found another potential tenant willing to pay 30% more for our place. If we didn't agree to pay the increased rate, we would need to move out within 30 days.

Naturally, my first reaction was, "WTF, lady?!?! How could you do this to us?" Luckily, my open-minded husband quickly swooped in with comforting words. "Maybe this is a good thing. I mean if you could do ANYTHING, and go ANYWHERE, what would you do?" I loved it when we balanced each other out like this. One mind going cray cray while the other mind pulls it back in.

I took in his question; it was an opportunity to dream big. "Well, I would move to Living Waters and make it into a thriving business. We could use our background in wellness, my experience in advertising, and offer yoga, Thai massage, and retreats to guests. I could paint and hang my artwork inside of the accommodations. You'd have time to write music. We could be surrounded by nature and live the slow-paced life we've always imagined. Wait a minute, we could actually GET PAID to live it!"

"Let's do it," he responded.

We sent an email to the owners pitching both ourselves and the business idea. *What's the worst that could happen? They could say "no" and we'd still be in the same boat: living in Dallas looking for our next home.*

Holy amazeballs! They actually said YES. Within three weeks, we were living at the property just in time to celebrate my 30th birthday.

The funny thing is that our landlord's new renter fell through, so she invited us to stay without the increase in rent. We declined.

THANK YOU, Ms. Landlord Lady, for helping us live our dreams. Without that extra kick in the butt, we may never have had the willingness to go within, get clear on what we wanted, and ask for it.

I logged this experience into my mental inventory as more proof that when "seemingly" shitty things happen, it can mean something even better is just around the corner. Maybe life really was always looking out for me.

I was astounded at how just asking myself this simple question, "*What if this is a good thing?*" could change my entire world. It actually *had* changed my entire world. It helped me test the theory I've heard from Byron Katie and many other spiritual teachers: *Life happens for me, not to me.* Not only was I discovering that this was true for me, I also got to see how life secretly prepares me for what is to come. It may sound airy-fairy, but I had solid evidence. Looking over my life, I found even more proof of this truth. Here are just a few examples:

I broke my ankle, which led me to meet my husband.

I burnt out in my advertising career, which led me to quit my job and move to Spain.

I failed my first yoga training, which led me to launch my career as a private yoga instructor.

I was at war with my parents, which led me to attend a Byron Katie event that forever changed my life.

I had years of intense migraines, which led me to learn how to make peace with pain and illness.

I became a Certified Facilitator for The Work of Byron Katie™, which led me to know exactly what to do to support myself in the biggest curveball yet: cancer.

Gosh! If only I could *always* remember this universal truth, that *life is for me*, in every moment. I'd sure as heck save a lot of time and avoid a lot of unnecessary suffering. This stubborn mind of mine tends to forget so darn quickly.

Our dream job of managing a B&B was quite an adventure, a beautiful and challenging and frustrating and healing one. Running a retreat property wasn't always a retreat for me. It was a ton of work, eventually leading to a ton of inner work.

It took some time to adjust to a lifestyle of being on-call around the clock and dealing with property issues such as high-maintenance guests, things constantly breaking at inopportune times (usually saved for my birthday, Valentine's Day, or when we were on vacation), monster storms demolishing the gardens and outdoor landscaping, Hill Country mice pooping everywhere, bridezillas, and that time a panicked guest called about the "dead animal" in his room, which turned out to be a dried-up wasp carcass. *OK, wait—that was just HILARIOUS!*

Working with my husband was…well, work. Our differences in working styles began to reveal themselves: me, the Type A Planner who liked to be organized, over-plan, over-think, and, yes, often over-stress about details in order to avoid disasters. Then there was my husband, Captain Last-Minute Man, who would choose to pot a plant when wedding guests were arriving in 30 minutes and the accommodations still weren't ready.

On top of everything else, we were commuting to and from Dallas to spend time with our precious six-year-old godson, Nainoa, whom we were helping raise. He lived with his grandmother, and we had hoped that they would join us in Austin. However, she decided to postpone her retirement and remain in

Dallas. Although we were disappointed at first, this did allow us to keep our work with our private clients in Dallas going when we visited him. And we could bring him out to Living Waters for long weekends of nature time, fort building, bone collecting, hiking, swimming, and dirt bike riding. It was the intimate family bonding time we had always imagined, the time and space to really enjoy and just be with each other.

However, over time the four-hour commute and the stress of my "dream job" began to weigh heavily on my mind and body. I turned to some not-so-healthy habits for dealing with stress, like that good ol' wine and TV. I just wanted to shut off my overactive mind that was constantly running with to-do lists, coordinating plans in two cities, worrying about guests' experiences, and harshly judging myself for not handling it all better. I couldn't even go for a walk on the beautiful grounds without seeing a billion projects that needed to be completed. My migraines were also getting out of control. Nearly half of the month was spent in intense pain.

I had already learned great tools for managing stress, like yoga, art, journaling, and inquiry-based meditation, but my practices of each became totally half-assed and inconsistent. I found myself in a difficult, yet familiar, place: unhappy.

It's truly fascinating to me that when it feels like life is taking a big dump on you, you find that those turds are actually fertilizer for personal growth. Sometimes I just have to go to what doesn't work and live in pain for a bit in order for a change to arise. Luckily, this girl has a low tolerance for suffering.

One day, I was sitting on the couch in our cozy pink cottage, watching an online interview with Byron Katie. I had been introduced to her practice of self-inquiry, called "The Work," a few years ago. The Work is a simple yet powerful process of identifying and questioning thoughts that create stress. It's a way to clear your mind and see that reality is actually pretty awesome.

Hearing Byron Katie (everyone calls her "Katie") speak with such clarity and peace brought back memories of when The Work was a daily practice in my life. I was moved to tears remembering the freedom I had previously felt. I paused the recording to contemplate…*Why did I stop doing The Work? And how can I get back on track?* My heart nearly leapt out of my chest when the thrilling decision hit: I'm signing up for the Certification Program in The Institute for The Work of Byron Katie. *Heck ya!*

Becoming a Certified Facilitator appealed to me as it was a natural (and pretty badass) compliment to my work as a yoga therapist, but that wasn't my main intention for joining. I did it to hold myself accountable for doing my own inner work through the various online classes, one-on-one work, and events with Katie and other Certified Facilitators. Yes, everything anyone needs to know to do The Work can be found on Byron Katie's website for free (freedom is free!), but I felt like my rigid mind needed a more structured boot camp.

What I loved most about the program was that it wasn't a training on how to *teach* The Work, it was a training on how to *live* The Work. How to take my yoga practice off the mat and into my life. How to stop resisting the challenges that life brings and meet them with an open, curious mind. How to actually live my favorite Gandhi quote: "Be the change you wish to see in the world."

The Work consists of four simple questions and some turnarounds. When you are feeling stressed, the invitation is to pause and notice what you're thinking and believing, write it down, and investigate its validity using inquiry.

The four questions are:

1. *Is it true?*
2. *Can you absolutely know that it's true?*
3. *How do you react, what happens, when you believe that thought?*
4. *Who would you be without that thought?*

The turnarounds are a way to examine the original stressful thought from different perspectives. They open the mind to seeing other possibilities in life—possibilities that we are blind to when we are under the influence of a stressful thought. (For a more in-depth explanation of the process, jump to the Appendix.)

Over the next two years at Living Waters, I immersed myself in the ultimate inner adventure of investigating my stressful stories around every frustrating part of my life.

My relentless mind was determined to find a stressful situation that was actually true, that was actually the reason for my suffering. Proof that the problem was out there, that it couldn't be solved from the inside. *Four questions that can change your life? Surely, it can't be this simple.*

Yet each time I brought my issues to inquiry, I discovered that it was my thinking about the situation, the person, or thing that was the problem. The problem was never out there. Not even once. Each time I was stressed, I was simply stuck in BS (belief systems). A cheesy rhyme, but totally true!

As my mind began to shift and change, I watched my husband transform before my eyes. Instead of wanting to strangle him, I fell in love with him all over again. By pushing my buttons, he taught me to come back home to myself, to reality. I began to see all of the ways that we actually did work well together, and I learned to appreciate our differences. Inquiry offered a stable support system for both of us within our marriage, a go-to place when we felt frustrated and triggered. Shockingly, this actually brought us back to how we felt when we first met. Perhaps the honeymoon phase is simply a state of mind that's always accessible.

I witnessed my job getting easier as my thoughts about my job started to unravel. The work and to-do lists living in my head were much bigger than they were in reality, and now I could appreciate the challenges and see how they were growing me. My job taught me how to stay present in the midst of apparent chaos, to creatively solve problems, and how to turn "work mode" off in my mind and enjoy the beauty around me. I was then able to experience the incredible bonuses of living on the property and running the business: the creativity, the connections with new people, the nature, the alone time, the romantic time, the stillness.

As I questioned my stressful stories about motherhood and parenting, I fell into a new, deep appreciation and connection with my godson, who became a son to me. He taught me how to see the world through a child's eyes, with excitement, wonder, and curiosity—and how to make *anything* fun.

I found relief from physical pain by questioning my stories about my migraines, thoughts like, *I have a migraine. It's getting worse. I want it to go away. I need to find the cure now!* I noticed how at the first sign of a migraine, my mind would jump to the past or future, but when I was present to the sensations and dropped my story about them, the pain would often dissipate. When I shifted my reaction to them, the pain shifted too. *So cool!* I began to see migraines as teachers, helping me learn how to slow down, be present, breathe, and stay in my yoga and inquiry practice.

My yoga also began to shift; I was able to meet my body without the recurring critical stories, and in turn, I began to fall in love with it. My body became a friend, a guide. In my yoga classes and retreats, I started to invite others to do the same, to notice the narratives we hold about our bodies, about life, and to observe how the body tenses up and loses its breath when we're under the influence of such stories. Who would we be without our body judgments? How would you stretch a hamstring without the story, "It should be different…more flexible, more open, it should look like hers"? Perhaps more relaxed, patient, and connected to your body, your practice. Now this was my kind of yoga, yo!

I became fascinated with life and with the intricacies of my mind. I witnessed the power of perception, that how I viewed the world created my experience of the world. A simple shift in perception could change everything! This peace was here inside of me, all along. It was just masked by a shitload of innocent, confused, stressful thoughts.

In 2015, I finished my training and became a Certified Facilitator, and my new passion of sharing Yoga & The Work could now be realized. My husband and I also wanted to be closer to Nainoa in Dallas so we could be a bigger part of his life, especially during his transition from childhood to adolescence. We really missed him.

It became increasingly clear that it was time to let the B&B go, and as life would have it, we found the perfect couple to take our place: my younger brother and future sister-in-law. They had just returned from a year of backpacking around the world and weren't ready for a 9-to-5 job. They were also already familiar with the property from our wedding retreat and from being hired as private chefs for my yoga retreats.

The summer of 2015 saw big transitions in our jobs, home, family life, and passions. I had been staffing Byron Katie events and led my very first international yoga retreat in Costa Rica. It was all coming together, my new life of Yoga & The Work. Oh, and my ego just loved that I was "the first" to do this, a true "pioneer." Oh boy. I developed a solid marketing brand and made plans to launch programs at several different yoga studios upon my return to Dallas. *Get ready, world!*

Life had different plans. Throughout all of these exciting transitions, my greatest yoga teacher, my guru, was silently growing inside of me, just waiting to be discovered.

Life is simple. Everything happens for you, not to you. Everything happens at exactly the right moment, neither too soon nor too late. You don't have to like it...it's just easier if you do.

—BYRON KATIE

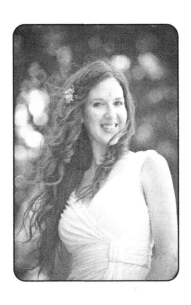

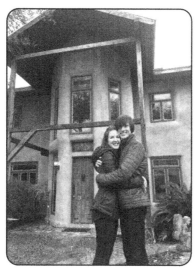

Living Waters on Lake Travis

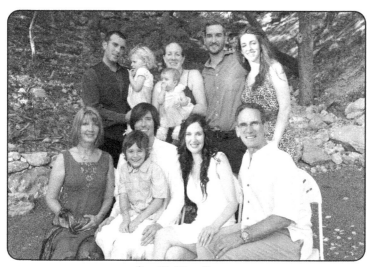

Our Wedding Retreat

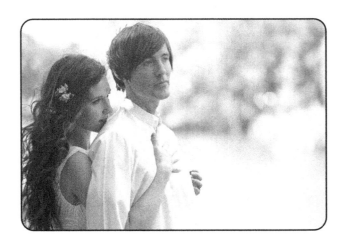

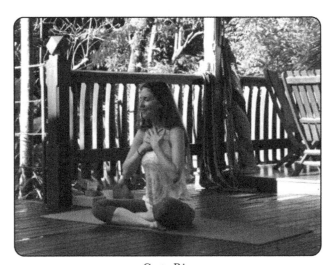

Costa Rica

2

My Lulus & My Love

JUST BEFORE THE SUMMER of awesomeness, I could feel the November breast lump starting to get bigger. Soon a lump the size of a golf ball appeared in my left armpit. *Hmmmmm... this is different.*

A friend and fellow yoga teacher whom I had met at Living Waters, Lonne, had just been diagnosed with an aggressive form of cancer, which had begun as a pain in her hamstring. *Hmmmmm... if healthy Lonne the Lioness can get cancer, maybe I'm not exempt after all.*

It was time to get those lumpies checked out.

Obviously, this yogini went the non-traditional healing route by seeing a naturopath for breast thermography. Breast thermography takes digital photos that measure the heat in the breast tissue. Since anything cancerous is inflammation, the heat of abnormalities will be visible via the color red on the images. The naturopath can then determine whether a lump is likely to be cancerous. Since the test does not involve radiation, it really appealed to me. I had done breast thermography on the very first lump I detected back in the day, and the results were congruent with those from my traditional medical doctors—just a swollen lymph node. So I trusted this process.

At my first session, I got the kickass news I'd been hoping for! The naturopath did not detect any signs of cancer in my breast or armpit. *Ahhhhh, sweet relief!* My estrogen did look a little elevated, however. He hypothesized that the lumps were likely swollen lymph nodes or cysts and sent me home with recommendations for lymphatic drainage therapy via a homeopathic tincture taken three times per day, three sessions of lymphatic drainage to stimulate and cleanse my lymphatic system, and a follow-up appointment six months later.

Despite my efforts to adhere to his plan, after six weeks, there was no change in the size of my lumps. In fact, they were expanding. I could even see one protruding from my breast. Confused and unsettled, I went back to the naturopath and underwent two more thermography sessions. Again, the results showed no signs of cancer.

Yet something still didn't feel right. When I asked him if I should seek out an ultrasound or mammogram to make sure there was nothing to worry about, he replied that it was up to me, but to remember that "mammograms cause cancer."

Geez, believing this thought was what had kept me from doing one in the first place, and here it was again. I began to wonder if perhaps mammograms weren't so bad after all. I told myself that maybe in rare cases they did cause cancer, but I had also heard that they were good at detecting it. Besides, his staff had already hooked up electrodes to my tumors to "flush" my lymphatic system. This sounds effective at first, but considering that you are flushing something that is full of cancer, it could be a great way to spread cancer to other locations in your body. If I had listened to his "come back in six months" advice, I might have been in a very different situation. As in…not alive…and not writing this book!

My inner voice finally got loud enough for me to comply: *Get another opinion, chica!* I said "peace out, naturopath."

Frantically, I started calling around to see if I could have an ultrasound somewhere in Dallas and get an estimate for the out-of-pocket cost. I felt frustrated, inconvenienced, and annoyed at the lack of a clear answer. Furthermore, I was pissed at myself for being uninsured, because times like these are the very reason why people get insurance—to find peace of mind in the face of unexpected events. My inner tape recorder was playing the word "idiot" on repeat, which never fails to make a stressful situation even more fun.

Then I found an angel in the form of a woman who had been in my life for eight years: my mother-in-law, Elaine. I knew she worked in a doctor's office, but had no idea what kind, and she jumped at the opportunity to support me. She quickly arranged an appointment for me with one of her nurses for a manual exam free of charge; the doctor could then refer me to a clinic for a mammogram and ultrasound.

During my manual exam, I learned that my lump was a little bigger than the typical ol' lump examined by doctors. The nurse's eyes nearly popped out of her head as I twisted to the right, exposing the bulge in the side of my breast. "Ummm…I'm going to get the head doctor. I'll be right back," she nervously said while maintaining a smile on her face and slowly walking backwards towards the door. *OK. Glad for the extra eyes, I guess?*

The doctor agreed that I needed to get it checked out ASAP. The good news was that the lump in my breast was not fixed (it was movable), so it still could have been a mere fibroadenoma. Still, she expressed concern at the fact that there was another lump hanging out in the armpit.

Angel Elaine made my appointment for the mammogram and ultrasound. I still had mixed feelings about mammograms and the radiation exposure. However, I had heard that the combination of these two tools together would be my best option for an accurate diagnosis of what was unfolding in my body. Plus, I found out that a mammo emitted the same amount of radiation that I would have received from flying on an airplane. That wouldn't stop me from flying, so why would I let it stop me from self-care? I tried to look at the mammo as simply a way to go from point A (unknown territory) to point B (more information).

After the doctor's visit, a little anxiety started to creep in. Anxiety is a signal that tells me to pause and notice what I'm thinking and believing and bring it to inquiry. *Something horrible is going to happen. These lumps are deadly cancer. My life is over!* After questioning these stressful thoughts, I could clearly see that it wasn't the lumps that were stressing me out. They were totally innocent balls of tissue hanging out in my body. It was the labels I was putting on them (*CANCER! I'M DYING!*) that were fueling my anxiety. It was time to come back to the present moment. The truth was (and is), everything was actually OK right here, right now.

And why not color a tough situation with a lil' humor? I decided to re-label my lumps with cute new names: Lulu 1 (breast lump) and Lulu 2 (armpit lump). This made me giggle and helped me to see them in a new light, as sweet and innocent. Now I could take my Lulus to get an ultrasound and mammogram. My new little buddies, my new little Buddhas.

Up to this point, I surprisingly hadn't experienced too much stress. I told myself that I'd save my big freak-out until there was something real to freak out about. Right now, the doctors were just making sure that all was good in my body. Unfortunately, this zen feeling didn't last too long.

Two days before the appointment, thoughts began to bombard me like a freight train. *I'm dying! I may not have a future with my husband like I thought.*

One evening, I was making love with Travis in our bedroom and was suddenly filled with a deep sadness. I gently propped myself up, placing my hands on his broad, comforting shoulders. As soon as I looked into his eyes, the emotions poured out of me. The moment didn't feel real; he didn't feel real. His realness was fading. There was deep, gut-wrenching sadness, yet it was accompanied by a subtle curiosity, a surrender, and an intense pleasure. I felt merged with him as my tears fell from my eyes onto his cheeks. His smile. This cosmic, beyond-this-world love, knowing we'd always be connected no matter what. I flashed to a similar experience I had had making love to him when we first met, this knowingness. We just laid in each other's arms and couldn't speak. It seemed that this "I might have cancer" experience was already re-shaping our relationship. There was a sweetness, a tenderness, a wordless appreciation for each other.

Images of our history filled my mind as if flipping through a catalogue of synchronistic love stories. We had met a little over eight years prior in a bookstore. This is so funny to me now, because a bookstore was the absolute last place I would have been during that time in my life. I was 25 and had been working as an account executive in a big, snazzy advertising agency in Dallas.

I had a work-hard, play-hard mentality and relished the constant activity and adrenaline of the advertising life that I had jumped into right after graduating from SMU. However, over time, this lifestyle started to wear on me. I began to notice a mental pattern of *I'll be happy when* _____. *I'll be happy when this project is over. After this business trip. When my salary increases. When I meet the right guy.*

I was always putting my happiness outside of me and way in the future. It dawned on me that I had the rest of my life to work my ass off, but this was the *only* time that I would be young and single with zero attachments. My bestie, who worked in finance, shared the same feelings. Daringly, we quit our jobs and bought one-way tickets to Barcelona, Spain. *Yeah, baby!*

Two months before leaving, I was partying with some work friends and competed in a "Flip Cup Tournament"—a ridiculous (OK, and really fun) drinking game that involves working as a team to chug beer and flip over red plastic cups. Our team was named "The Ducking Frunks" and we had matching shirts to prove it. Let's just say our team won…meaning we were the drunkest people at the party.

In pure excitement from our win (#lifeaccomplishments), I spontaneously jumped up on my friend's back for a celebratory piggyback ride. I forgot to inform him of my plans, and before I knew it, we both slammed down onto the floor. My right ankle broke our fall. Literally. There must have been a really loud noise, because the room fell silent as everyone stared in horror. I shook it off like everything was fine—a favorite coping mechanism of mine—and immediately stood up. My ankle wasn't having any of it, and it took me right back down to the floor. *Oh crap.*

Showing up to work with a cast and crutches that following Monday was…well…undeniably embarrassing. I really wanted to invent a new, more heartwarming story about how I broke it, like by jumping into the street to save a small boy from being hit by a car. *I'm a hero!* Nope. I had to hold my head high and wear that drunken shame like a badge of honor.

I remember experiencing so much frustration over not being able to do daily things, like drive a car or carry a cup of coffee to my desk. One day, I found myself in tears at the bottom of the hardwood stairs of my three-story townhouse. My girlfriend was about to pick me up for dinner, and I had finally gotten myself all ready, cute outfit on and crutches in hand. Then I looked down and noticed I had forgotten my damn shoe. I glanced up at the stairs, a gazillion wooden steps towering above me. I totally lost it like a two-year-old girl told that she can't have that pony. *Why me?!!! It's not fairrrrrrrr!* My friend immediately tried to console me after she walked through the door to find me in a pool of pitiful tears. "It's ok, I'll go get your shoe!"

It wasn't about the shoe. For the first time in a long time, I was forced to depend on other people. I had to endure the vulnerability of asking for help. It made me cringe. This independent, career-driven, perfectionist lady did not like it one bit!

Yet once I finally gave into this inevitable lesson, it opened my eyes to seeing how people are *always* willing to help. It actually feels really good to help someone in need. If I'm totally honest with myself, it also feels good to stop trying to be in control all of the time and to receive support from others.

My mom flew out to help me too, because that's what many mothers of 25-year-old adults do. And this time I gratefully accepted the assistance. She chauffeured me, took me to my appointment to get a stylish giant ankle boot, and stocked my freezer full of homemade chicken noodle soup. We even managed to have a fun night out, sipping chocolate martinis on the glass rooftop patio of Ghost Bar in the W Hotel. We may have used my "medical condition" as a way to bypass the long line of trendy Dallas uptowners. *Perhaps there are a few perks here after all!*

At home one evening while I was once again consumed by self-pity (yes, I'll admit it—I was a bit of a drama queen), Mom tenderly asked, "How do you know something good won't come from this? Maybe you'll meet the man of your dreams because he's holding the door open for you or something."

Well, it wasn't a door. It was a stool. Two weeks later, on May 1st, I walked into a bookstore to buy my younger brother a book about New York City, where he'd be interning at the Guggenheim over the summer. I almost didn't go in because the store looked closed. Standing in the travel section, I heard a man's voice. "Excuse me, I saw your ankle and thought you might want this." I looked over to see a stool in his hand.

"Oh, thank you!" I responded.

"So...are you traveling somewhere?" he asked.

I glanced up to see his dazzling green eyes on the other side of the bookshelf. *Damn, he's cute.* We started to talk about our travels, my brother's internship in New York, my trip to Spain, and his desire to visit Costa Rica.

After talking for a while, I made the courageous decision to walk over to his side of the bookshelf, confirming my suspicion that this guy was HAWT! Beyond looks, there was something so intriguing about him. He was different than the usual guy I was attracted to; he wasn't a frat guy or a cowboy.

He politely excused himself to take a quick phone call. "Hey man, yeah I'm at the bookstore. You can head over to my place and I'll meet you there. Jenny's home."

Wait—what? This guy has a live-in girlfriend? You've got to be kidding me! Again, more proof guys suck. I can't wait to get my ass to Spain.

"No, she just barks a lot, she won't bite you." *OMG–Jenny's a dog! Jenny's a dog! Woohoo!*

I kept my cool as he hung up the phone. We continued to flirt for about an hour, and he asked me what types of therapies I was doing to heal my ankle. I responded with, well, nothing, and he offered me some Reiki and acupressure to help it heal faster.

I had no idea what that meant. All I heard was "hot guy wants to touch me," so obviously, I accepted. The very next day, we had an ankle massage date at my place.

I couldn't remember his name, so I dubbed him "Borders," the name of the bookstore, in my flip phone. I'll never forget the bewildered look on my roommate's face when I told him, "Hey, there's a hot guy that I met last night at the Borders bookstore. He's coming over to massage my ankle. I don't remember his name, so if you could just introduce yourself and get his name... that would be swell. Cool?"

The next day we learned this glorious man did have a name: Travis.

As a side note on names, the biblical meaning of Travis is "a crossing into." Bethany translates to "house of God," so I guess that together we were crossing into the house of God. For me, our relationship was the start of a spiritual awakening on all levels, physically, mentally, emotionally, and oh my...definitely sexually.

We were practically inseparable for the next two months as I transitioned out of my advertising job and prepared for Spain. He came to Florida to meet my parents. We vacationed on Captiva Island, where we may have had sex nine times in one day. He flew out to NYC to be with me before my flight left for Europe. As cliché as it may sound, it truly was a real-life whirlwind romance novel.

I knew I loved him, yet I somehow remained unattached to the outcome. If it was meant to be, it would be. I loved that he supported my travels, but my body felt otherwise and ached for him…I'll never forget the nauseating pit in my stomach when we hugged and kissed goodbye at the JFK airport. It was physically painful to let him go. I vowed to myself that I wouldn't call him for a while—I wasn't going to be "that girl." My resolve lasted for about a week. Love just couldn't resist making contact. I wanted to share everything with him, and soon we were talking multiple times per day.

After I'd been living in Spain for a month, he came to visit. We traveled up and down the Spanish coastline before flying to Cinque Terre, Italy, for ten days.

Cinque Terre is a group of five tiny fishing villages on the stunning Mediterranean coast of Italy. I had been once before when I studied abroad in Paris during my junior year of college. My girlfriends and I had hopped on a train from Florence for a day hike to one of the villages, Monterosso. When my eyes first set sight on that bright turquoise ocean crashing into the gorgeous jagged cliffs at sunset, my first thought was, "This is where I'm honeymooning with my future husband."

Apparently Travis and I had silently decided to skip the courting and the wedding and go straight for that honeymoon. We spent our days lying on the beach feeding each other freshly picked blackberries, swimming and making out in the cool, crystal-clear water. After our afternoon nap and lovemaking, we'd hop from town to town on the train to sip local wines and devour pizza, pasta, and tomato caprese to our hearts' desire.

One evening, we found ourselves dining at the upscale Restaurante Miky in Monterosso. A giant, colorful, steaming pot of salty seafood paella had just been delivered to our table when I looked him straight in the eyes and daringly stated, "I'm going to marry you. You know that, right?" I had never felt so confident, so free to be this honest with a man before.

"Yes, I know." He matter-of-factly confirmed as his gentle fingertips seductively brushed over my hand. It was one of those timeless, slow-motion romantic movie moments where everything in the background fades away. Shivers went down my spine. There was no doubt in my mind: *this is it.*

The climax (pun intended) of the trip was a sunset hike through the last town, Riomaggiore. Pink, orange, and purple hues streaked across the expansive, blue sky. Huddled under a soft, red, butterfly sarong, we made love on top of a magnificent cliff overlooking the Mediterranean Sea. Our ears were filled with the background music of crashing waves, and our senses heightened by the exhilarating possibility of getting caught. I thought to myself, *seriously, is this really happening?*

After the most epic and romantic month of my life, Travis returned to Dallas. My heart hurt all over again. I remember thinking that this had to be the last time I was going to say a goodbye like this to him. To make my situation even more difficult, the girlfriend I had moved to Spain with had also decided she needed to head back home.

Yet I knew I was meant to be in Europe a little longer. So I stayed. It was an absolutely incredible time of self-healing and self-reflection. Unexpectedly, especially considering that I was in Europe, I decided to take a break from drinking alcohol. It felt like my body started to completely reject it. I would have one glass of wine and pay for it with a crazy hangover for three days. It just wasn't worth it while living in Barcelona. I discovered that *oh my God*…mornings *do* exist! I had more time, more spending money, and my body started feeling better.

Abstaining from drinking gave me the space to contemplate who I was without alcohol. It had been such an integral part of my social life for years that I had been blind to how much I was locked into the identity of being the fun party girl. I got curious about what I had thought alcohol was giving me in my life: fun, spontaneity, more ease in social situations, a way to be present. Then I looked for ways I could give myself these same experiences without alcohol (and thus without the hangover).

Being too cheap to buy a gym membership, I started doing my own yoga practice. I found a connection beyond the physical benefits, a sense of stillness, calmness, and inspiration. I started to teach it in Park Güell to some of my friends, which surprisingly felt extremely natural and fun.

I can't explain why, but I stopped eating meat as well. Meat just sounded disgusting. Maybe it was the pig carcasses that hung from the ceilings of every Spanish restaurant and market. My meals became plant-based and organic, full of color and dense in nutrients. I didn't have this language at the time, but now I see that my body was going through some type of deep cleansing process.

I began traveling by myself, something I had never done before because I had been too afraid. I'll never forget sitting on the bus for my first solo trip to Budapest and hearing Celine Dion's song "All by Myself" bust out over the speakers. I laughed out loud as a tear trickled down my cheek. From Budapest to Vienna, I couchsurfed at stranger's homes. Even though I met fascinating people, I still preferred to spend the majority of my time on my own. I had finally found the perfect travel mate: me.

During that time, I reconnected with my creative side and started to journal and draw again as I had when I was a child. My last apartment in Barcelona featured a five-foot balcony overlooking Antoni Gaudi's famous church, La Sagrada Familia. It was so close by that I could actually hear the daily construction of this iconic gothic cathedral that looks like it was engineered with hot wax candle drippings. Every day, I sat on that tiny, concrete balcony in my vintage foldout chair, pen and journal in hand, and stared at the world with curiosity and wonder. I'd watch the wrinkly local elders joyfully play bocce ball, take in the scent of garlic and onions from neighboring restaurants, and would free-flow write for hours. For the first time, I truly enjoyed silence and solitude. Admittedly, my homebody tendencies were likely enhanced by the 90 steep steps up to that apartment door. At least my ankle had healed!

It was a time of learning that I am enough, that I can do anything, that I am free. I had to find me first. Even though I hadn't read the book yet, I had unknowingly *Eat, Pray, Love*'d the shit out of my life. After five months in Barcelona, I took this mindset back to the States. One week later, on New Year's Eve, while sitting in a candle-lit spiral of rose petals on the beach of St. Petersburg, Florida, Travis proposed to me.

Isn't it marvelous to discover that you're the one you've been waiting for? That you are your own freedom?

—BYRON KATIE

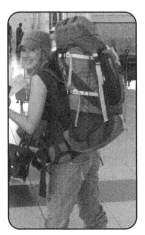

Off to Spain

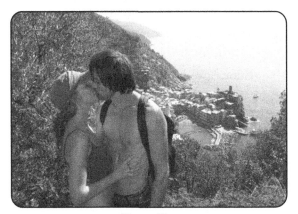

Cinque Terre

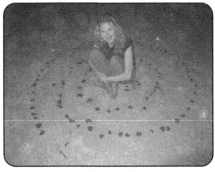

Engaged!

3

How I Found Peace During "The Waiting Game"

A STARK SILENCE FILLED THE AIR as Travis and I drove to my appointment for the mammogram and ultrasound. We pulled into the parking lot and I turned to look at the strip mall in front of me. The diagnostic facility was right next to one of our favorite Asian restaurants. Never during any of those meals did I imagine that one day I'd be getting tested for cancer right next door. *I already miss my old life.*

"I can't believe that we will be leaving this building knowing whether or not I have cancer. This is so crazy!" I said as Travis locked the car and reached for my hand.

"I'm here for you honey, it will be OK." His words comforted me.

My heart began to race, my first experience of what cancer patients call scanxiety. My mind couldn't help but jump into a scary future. I struggled to focus on breathing and being in the present moment.

A door swung open. "Bethany, we are ready for you now."

In a small room, I sat down near a mysterious, big-ass silver machine. The technician was an incredibly gentle, plump lady who was definitely someone's loving grandmother. She walked me through the process. First, disrobe and put on the sexy floral, baby blue hospital gown (which had a giant tear in it). Second, put little stickers with metal in them over my moles and freckles so that the radiologist could distinguish them from internal lumps on the mammogram. She informed me that all of the young girls in the office liked to take them home and put them on their nipples for their boyfriends. *Lol, I'll pass.* Thirdly, place my boob in the ginormous machine with a pancake-smashing device that would squash me several times from several angles.

If there's anything that can suck the sexiness out of young, voluptuous 34DD boobies, it's the mammo. *Dear God, I had no idea they could be contorted like this.*

My boob finally somehow made it into the George Foreman. As soon as I heard a buzzing noise, she told me in a calm, soothing voice, "DON'T breathe." The machine snapped the image. "You CAN breathe." Boob got smashed from a new angle. "DON'T breathe." Snap. "You CAN breathe." This continued until she looked satisfied with the quantity of images.

In all honesty, it wasn't as painful or as horrible as I had thought. Of course, during the entire process, I studied the shit out of the technician's face as she looked at my images…trying to distinguish some facial expression, a twitch, a frown, any sign that would let me know what was growing in my boob. But she was a master of the poker face, shining her cheery grandma smile the whole time.

After the mammogram, she explained that she would show the images to the radiologist who could then determine if an ultrasound was necessary. She looked at me with a reassuring smile, saying, "I am almost positive that... (*Oh good! She's going to say there's nothing to worry about!*) ...that you'll also need an ultrasound. Be right back!" *Dammit.*

Ten minutes later, she entered the room, extremely smiley and chipper. "I have good news!" (*Oh goodie! It's not cancer!!!*) and finished her sentence with, "You'll DEFINITELY need an ultrasound!"

Seriously? This lady really needed a crash course in how to deliver news to patients. Then again, this woman was living in reality. The reality that reality is GOOD. No matter what. So I brushed off my irritation as I headed into the ultrasound room.

After the cold and goopy ultrasound, the new technician asked if I wanted anyone with me when the doctor gave me the results. I asked her to please fetch my husband from the waiting room. "He'll be easy to find, he's the really cute guy." She responded, "Oh, I think I already spotted him. Brown hair?" *That's my baby!*

Travis's face was so sweet when he walked in, full of so much love and concern, saying "Honey, are you OK?" as he rushed to me. I explained that I didn't have any news yet and just wanted him to be with me when I heard. The radiologist and technician returned, requesting another ultrasound and a few more minutes of looking at the images.

Oh God, this is it.

She sat down on a stool, took a deep breath, and faced me. Time froze. She looked me in the eyes and said that since my breast tissue was so dense, she was unable to determine with certainty what the lumps were. They could be cancerous, benign, or a simple infection. A biopsy of both the breast and armpit area would tell us for sure.

All of my "not too much stressness" took a total exit stage left at this moment. *What. The. Fuck. I just went through all of that for nothing? You STILL don't know? I HAVE to WAIT even longer?! I was supposed to know TODAY. She should be able to diagnose me. I want her to tell me NOW!* And the tears and fear started to pour out.

My husband said, "Honey, this is great news. She is not saying you have cancer." But I couldn't hear a word. I was consumed by pure frustration.

We left that building stuck in the same damn place: the land of the unknown. I called my parents crying as Travis picked up chicken noodle soup from Whole Foods. Screw no meat and gluten! I wanted my childhood comfort food for an evening full of self-pity.

The next day, I had an appointment with my primary care doctor. She explained the situation again, and we talked about how it would be a really good time to get health insurance. Amid her apologies and words about how I was too young to have to go through something like this, I realized that this was all starting to sound way too real for me. Could it really be possible that I had cancer? I was young. I was healthy. I lived a really healthy lifestyle. I freaking taught "wellness" for a living! There was no history of breast cancer in my family. How could this be possible?

When I got home, I started diving into questioning my stressful thoughts using The Work. I wrote a Judge-Your-Neighbor (or in my case Judge-Your-Doctor) Worksheet about the moment when the radiologist shared the news (or lack thereof). A Judge-Your-Neighbor Worksheet is a free tool available on Byron Katie's website that helps you identify and collect stressful thoughts so you can then take them to inquiry. It's a great way to mentally vomit all of your frustrations, without censorship, and mine usually include a few (OK, let's be honest—a shitload of) cuss words. This exercise always gives my ego a landing place, a safe home to be expressed. And then to be investigated.

Through inquiry, I caught up with the reality that this really was good news. The radiologist was NOT telling me I had cancer. She cared enough to look me in the eyes, face me, and share her desire to have more testing done so we could get a clear picture of what was going on in my body. Not a guess. That's what I wanted too. We were on the same team. My anger towards her completely faded away; I could that see she was doing the best she could with the information available.

Not knowing at this moment was actually good for me. This extra time gave me more space to process, inquire, and mentally prepare for possibilities. I made the many phone calls required to get full health insurance coverage that would start in one month. Thankfully, because we had just moved back to Dallas, we qualified for a special enrollment period with Obamacare. I know people talk a lot of smack about the Affordable Care Act, but not me. Obama is seriously my hero.

After getting an out-of-pocket quote of $825 for the biopsy, I decided to schedule it ASAP instead of waiting for my insurance to kick in. For my mental peace, it was worth every penny to address this as soon as possible.

I tried to focus my mind on other fun things in life, like my 34th birthday the following week. *Woot! Woot!* I had parties, my husband's music gig, and lunch dates coming up. Oh, yeah, and maybe cancer.

So to recap, I had already cultivated quite the magical healing toolbox for handling stress. In fact, it felt like I had unknowingly been preparing for this situation my entire life. Thanks to these skills, I immediately dropped into a state of unwavering peace and gratitude.

Just kidding! Nope. At first, I threw every single tool of peace out the window (again) and turned to the art of freaking out, ugly crying, self-pity, and depression. I was a crazy, emotional hot mess. Out of nowhere, I would just curl into a ball and cry for hours.

One low point involved my extremely loving, well-intentioned mother sending me a 700-page book titled *Dr. Susan Love's Breast Book* subtitled *The bible for women with breast cancer*. I know she meant well, wanting to educate me and help put my mind at ease. (Later, I would discover this was one of THE most helpful resources! Mother's intuition again?)

I opened the book. All it took was reading the chapter headings for me to totally lose it. A volcano of uncontrollable emotions erupted from me. Anger. Frustration. Fear. Depression. Anxiety. I felt like a helpless little girl, all alone in the world. A victim of a cruel universe that didn't give a shit about me.

My mind was consumed with painful stories: *I definitely have cancer! Cancer will make my life more difficult. I shouldn't be so upset. I need the test results NOW. I don't know what to do.*

In fact, I did "know" what to do with these stressful thoughts—question them—but there were just too many flooding in. All I really wanted to do was crawl into a dark cave, be alone, and cry. So that's exactly what I did.

It's easy to be spiritual when things are going your way.

—BYRON KATIE

After I came to the realization that suffering sucks ass, I finally found the courage and motivation to call the Do The Work Helpline, a free service available to anyone who is experiencing stress. Volunteers on the helpline are extremely experienced in The Work and can facilitate inquiry for callers, answer questions about The Work, assist callers in identifying stressful thoughts, and share their own experience of inquiry. I had served on the helpline myself as a part of the training program, and I continued to do so.

I noticed unease at being on the other end of the phone line, feeling that somehow calling the helpline would reveal me as a failure at doing my own work and not living up to the high Certified Facilitator standard I had invented in my mind. As soon as I admitted this to myself, I was immediately met with *That's just bullshit, Bethany, call anyway!*

So I called. And then I called again. And again. The volunteers were so helpful and supportive as each call was met with gentle, non-judgmental, and nurturing voices on the other line. They held me in a compassionate and safe space of silence for my tears as they walked me through the four simple questions and turnarounds.

I experienced so much relief, so quickly, from these phone calls, that I was motivated to continue doing The Work on my own through writing. Writing out my answers is my favorite way to self-facilitate—if I try to do it in my head, inquiry takes ten times longer since my slippery ego constantly distracts me. *Is it true? What's for dinner?*

I had no shortage of stressful beliefs, that's for sure, and little by little, my anxiety and fear began to dissipate as I met each thought with understanding. Through inquiry, I discovered that I couldn't absolutely know that it was true that I had cancer. There was no solid evidence that cancer existed in my body. The only place it did exist is in my head, in my thinking. And are thoughts real? Can I feel, touch, and hold them? No. They are imagination.

How do I react, what happens when I believe these thoughts (Question 3)? The cancer in my mind spread like wildfire, painting a scary doomsday of a future. I saw images of my frail body in a hospital bed, dying, in unbelievable pain. Gray skin, no hair, no boobs. I had grown quite fond of my hair and boobs, considering them my greatest physical assets. In my mind they were now GONE FOREVER!

I saw images of saying goodbye to my husband, medical bills piling up, not knowing what to do, stress on my family and loved ones, no more travel, no more career that I love…dying young and becoming that "sad story" people talk about. The "I hope that never happens to me" story.

These thoughts hit me physically too. My shoulders, neck, head, and jaw tensed. I had headaches. My chest was caving in. I felt lethargic and didn't want to move. My daily walks and yoga practice fell to the wayside. I became cautious around my husband, not wanting to impose or ask too much. Around family, I acted as if everything was great, afraid to reveal my fears. I refrained from announcing what was happening to friends, embarrassed that I was making such a "big deal" without a diagnosis. A dark, heavy cloud settled over me.

Everything hung on the diagnosis: *if it's benign, I will be happy and free. If it's malignant, I am screwed.* I became a powerless victim.

I obsessed over trying to figure out HOW I got cancer—was

it my cell phone, this face soap, or the Vitamin D supplements I had been taking? I began to turn on myself, believing that I had surely done something wrong to deserve cancer. *I shouldn't have drunk so much in my early twenties. I could have been healthier, better, more perfect. If only I worked harder on healing myself or if I was more spiritual, this wouldn't be happening to me. God is punishing me.* I became angry at myself for getting angry, sad at my sadness. These thoughts felt so consuming, so powerful. In summary, when I believed my thoughts, it felt like SHIT.

As I sat in meditation on *Who would I be without these stressful thoughts? (Question 4)*, my entire experience eventually shifted. I felt lighter. My heart and mind opened. My body softened. I felt a sense of simplicity in this process…how well I had been following the simple instructions: Feel lump. Visit doctor. Get mammo/ultrasound. Schedule biopsy. Get insurance. Next step…next…next…I was not even the one doing it. I was being led.

I noticed that right here, right now, I was healthy, in amazing shape, thriving. I had more energy for walking and yoga. During my yoga practice, I gently caressed my Lulus and told them I loved them and was here to listen and learn from them. My witty sense of humor returned, including my cancer jokes (which not everyone appreciated BTW…learning!).

A little peace about the idea of having cancer crept in as I looked at how much I was discovering about myself, about life. *What if cancer is a wise teacher who is here to help me?* Without my thoughts, emotions were allowed to flow through me and didn't need a name. I remembered all of the remarkable people who had already lined up to support me, how I knew exactly what I needed to do in this moment: nothing. Reality was good. It was so simple. There was even a sense of inspiration about diving into the unknown. Getting the results even seemed exciting. *Whoa—did I just say that?*

The diagnosis transformed from a doomed death sentence into a new direction.

After getting a taste of life without my cancerous thinking (i.e., a taste of reality), I was inspired to investigate my desired outcome for tomorrow's biopsy: *I want the doctors to tell me I don't have cancer.* I held the moment of an imagined future in my mind: when the doctor called me with the biopsy results. My biggest insights appeared in the turnarounds.

First I turned it around to myself, *I want me to tell me I don't have cancer.* Well, geez, I wanted this from me right now, why wait until the phone call!? *It's TRUE!* I wanted me to remind myself that there was 100% absolutely no proof that I had one cancer cell in my body. How did I know? Nobody had told me. The tests hadn't proved it. There was no family history.

Even if the doctors did tell me that I have cancer, could I really know it was true in that moment? No, I couldn't. They were looking at scans, which are images of the past, and my body could have changed since then. Plus, tests have been wrong before.

Yet, I could still follow the simple instructions of the experts— more testing, the surgery, no surgery, chemo, no chemo. Even if part of my body did have cancer cells, the percentage of my body that had cancer would be miniscule. Let's say it was 8-10cm of tumors. OK, but what about the rest of me? *The majority of my body quite literally doesn't have cancer. Ummm, that's cool to know!*

I wanted me to tell me that I didn't have cancer because "I" can never have cancer. *I am not this body, I am so much more. Cancer can't touch my joy, my love for my family, my morning sip of tea, my walks in the park, my giggles, my tenacious spirit.* I could watch this body go through cancer and be here and support it in every possible way.

Flipping the thought to its opposite, *I want the doctors to tell me I have cancer. Oh shit, this turnaround is scary,* I noticed my superstitious ego coming in, saying, "Don't even think it...that's how you create cancer!" as if the mere words could change my Lulus from benign to malignant. I reminded myself to trust the process of The Work. How could this turnaround be true?

I wanted them to tell me I had cancer if it was true. I didn't want them to lie to me; instead I wanted them to use their years and years of medical training to tell me very clearly what they thought was going on in my body and how they recommended I handle it. I wanted pure honesty.

I wanted them to tell me because then I would know. I would have a clear direction as to where to go from here instead of being stuck in the "unknown" territory of waiting.

I wanted the doctors to tell me I had cancer so I could continue to question my thoughts about cancer. I was already realizing that cancer wasn't the problem—it was what I believed about Cancer (with a capital C!) that was scaring me in this moment. *What if the reality of cancer isn't so bad? What if it is good? What if it improves my life? How will I know unless I fully experience it?* So far, the only nightmares had been in my thinking...what if that was true throughout the entire process?

I wanted them to tell me so I could see that aside from what I was thinking and believing, I was still OK in this moment, learning the ultimate practice of presence.

I had already seen my relationship with my husband deepen. I could see us giggling in hospital beds, watching tons of movies, telling each other how much we love and appreciate each other. How did I know? This was happening with even the suggestion that I might have cancer! No more petty arguments, a renewed focus on what really matters. Perhaps all of my relationships would deepen.

My family would come visit me more....*ha!* I was usually

the one going to them. Still, I could see myself cherishing the moments with each one of them.

My career could shift into helping others cope with cancer. I would have so much compassion and be truly able to connect, saying "I have been here too." *This could be amazing!* Perhaps I was meant to get cancer so I could show the world what I am learning now, that cancer is not the "cancer" you think it is—it is a slowing down, self-care, connections, meaningful moments, appreciation, gratitude, humor. It's a teacher, a gift.

I wanted them to tell me I have cancer so I could explore the relationship between physical pain and the mind. I remembered what I came to realize with migraines: that my mind created more pain than existed in reality. *The intense pain was an illusion there—could it be the same in cancer treatment? What if I felt even better because of cancer treatment? What if it reset my body in some way so that my migraines disappeared?*

Maybe I would meet people on this path who would play important roles in my life forever, like doctors, caretakers, cancer survivors…new friendships and connections.

This inquiry was a complete game changer for me. Unbelievably, I felt the joy of a small child along with excitement for the next step—the next day's biopsy—and to discover where my life would lead. Past stressful experiences that had turned out to be good began to reenter my awareness: the broken ankle, failed yoga training, the mean landlord, challenging jobs.

Suddenly my case of the scary "What-ifs": *What if it's cancer… what if I'm dying…what if life is over…what if this is the WORST thing that could happen to me?* transformed into the exciting "What -ifs": *Yes, what if it IS cancer…what if I'm truly living…what if life is beginning…what if this is the BEST thing that could happen to me?"*

I mean, if I was going to live in an imaginary future anyways, why not choose one that felt good? And spoiler alert: Every. Single. Gift I anticipated actually did come to me. This was just the beginning of freedom from cancer.

It is easy to be swept away by some overwhelming feeling, so it's helpful to remember that any stressful feeling is like a compassionate alarm clock that says, "You're caught in the dream." Depression, pain, and fear are gifts that say, "Sweetheart, take a look at your thinking right now. You're living in a story that isn't true for you."

—BYRON KATIE

4

Diagnostic Testing
Without Stressing

BIOPSY DAY ARRIVED, and I was delighted to discover that I continued to feel this joy, openness, excitement, and detachment about the outcome. After a few morning yoga clients, I grabbed a quick veggie wrap and met my husband at home so we could ride together.

The whole process was so interesting to me. I became a witness to it all. Driving up to the hospital and seeing the big blue "Building 3: Cancer Center" sign, the adorable brunette who checked me in, the paperwork that allowed me to be treated, the sonogram lady named "Joy" who thoughtfully walked me through every step of the process as she took more ultrasound photos.

I was wearing comfortable black-and-white patterned floral, flowy pants with my hospital gown and had brought large cozy socks so my feet wouldn't get cold. Joy even offered me a warm blanket. *How amazing is that?* I felt the support of the soft hospital bed beneath me, the quiet atmosphere, the wealth of information being shared.

I began to feel a little nervous about the level of pain involved, so when Joy left to fetch the doctor who would be performing my biopsies, I used the time to quickly question the thought *It will be painful. Can I absolutely know it's true? The truth is…no, I can't know it—I've never experienced it. Zero proof. Zilch. Nada. Without the thought, I'm much more at ease, open, ready…Let's do this.*

I didn't feel a need to pretend myself beyond my evolution—I made sure to tell the doctors that I preferred to NOT see the massive needle or watch any of the procedure on the screen. *No thank you!* They thoughtfully offered to put a soft towel over my eyes. *Perfect.*

The procedure was less painful and much shorter than I had expected. There was a lovely large POP sound after each sample was sucked out from the needle. Lots of deep breathing. One of the holes bled more than usual, so I enjoyed the extra support of Joy applying a compress to it, then the doctor, then a stranger who walked in. *Wow, three doctors to one patient. I like this ratio.*

Everyone was so kind. They were surprised at how well I was doing (me too!), and I shared with them the inner work I had been exploring. The doctor commented, "Wow, you can really help others with this practice you're doing." *Hmmmm…maybe I will.* She especially loved hearing how I now saw a diagnosis as a new direction instead of a death sentence.

They wrapped my boobs up into a tight cocoon with ice packs tucked inside, somehow giving me both upper AND lower cleavage. After being briefed on how to take care of the wounds, how long to rest, and to take Tylenol if needed for any pain, I was informed that the results would arrive that week. And just like that, it was over.

My husband drove me home; we watched movies all day and ate yummy food. At this point, we had gone full-on organic and vegan. No more caffeine, sugar, alcohol, meat, dairy, gluten, or soy. Some people may feel this way of eating is restrictive, but for me it felt like a natural act of kindness to myself and my body. It was also helpful to remind myself to stay present. This was how I felt called to eat for the time being—not necessarily forever.

Over the next few days, I was honestly expecting fear and stress to arrive, but they never knocked on my door. I was blown away by this shift in perspective. *This is amazing!* I was so excited for the phone call, feeling at peace both with and without a diagnosis of cancer. Each path had its own beauty, meaning I could be happy now instead of waiting until I got the news. I was still open to experiencing that deep sadness and fear again, since it could happen, and I loved knowing how I would be there for myself in that too.

Being fearless didn't stop me from obsessively checking my cell phone a billion times over the next week. With every ring, my mind would immediately jump to, "Is this THE CALL that will determine my future?"

It was odd. I felt this excited, anxious anticipation. The same feeling I used to get right before a big basketball game in high school while I waited in the locker room, hearing cheering fans and 90's pop blasting in the gym. Or the adrenaline rush before starting one of my yoga retreats, staring at the front door ready for our first guest to appear.

Luckily, on Wednesday, September 16th, aside from teaching a morning yoga class, the rest of the day was open. I considered going to get my car washed, but decided to stay home instead, one eye watching my Netflix therapy and the other stalking my phone. When my sweetheart came home, he joined me on the couch. I was pretty confident the L-shaped cushion was already starting to form a permanent mold of my butt.

The phone rang. The screen glowed with the phone number for the PCP's office. We looked at each other as we held our breath. *Holy shit! This is it! Thank God I didn't go for that car wash!* The house went quiet as I answered the phone on speaker. We hovered over it, foreheads touching.

The doctor had just received the pathology report and wanted to call me as soon as possible. "This is the part of my job that's really difficult. I'm afraid I have bad news. They did find cancer in both the breast and lymph node."

Time stopped. Stillness felt. It was as if someone else's life was being described to me. I was a witness to each nanosecond of the moment. My hand grabbed Travis's hand.

"It's called invasive ductal carcinoma, grade 3, and it's the most common form of breast cancer."

Good—this means doctors will know how to deal with it. She shared how she recently had a patient who was 27 years old and diagnosed with the same cancer. She was now doing great and had just given birth to her first baby. "People make it through this and live very happy lives." *Wow, I love hearing this. She is so kind.*

She said she would send the pathology report to the breast surgeon—the steward of cancer treatment—so I could book my next appointment. Unfortunately, it is impossible to confirm the stage of the cancer from my biopsies or if it had spread to other areas. All we knew at this point was that it had started in my left breast, then metastasized into the lymph nodes in my left armpit.

My Lulus have cancer. I looked down at my breast. *Really? It looks so fine, it feels so fine other than some soreness from the biopsy. That's cancer in there? How is this possible?* As soon as I got off the phone, I turned to my husband. "What. What do I do next?" My mind struggled to jump into planning mode before the reality could sink in.

"Come here." He pulled me into his arms. The tears began to flow. The best words I can use to describe how I felt are "surreal" and "fucking weird." I loved how tightly he cradled me as we both cried and trembled together. My heart could have burst from my love for him. This moment remains one of my most favorite, most intimate experiences with him.

Then all of a sudden, my body became extremely hot. So hot, in fact, that I had to take off my tank top. I paced around the living room in my sports bra. *Wow. What? Really?* I literally pinched my arm multiple times to see if this was some sort of crazy dream. *Me? Cancer? Reallllllly?*

I Facetimed my mom. This part was really, really hard. Nobody wants to get this phone call from their child, and seeing the tears in my mother's soft hazel eyes while I told her the news made it more real. She nodded, "OK, OK."

Gratefully, the moment I asked her if she could come to Dallas, she responded immediately, "Yes, of course." She had already set the time aside just in case; her ticket was booked within an hour for a flight arriving the next day. We agreed that she would call my dad while I notified my two brothers.

What was plaguing my mind the most was HOW and WHY? *HOW did "I" get cancer? WHY did I get cancer, especially at such a young age?* I thought that perhaps all of the inner work I had done leading up to this point would have given me a "cancer bypass." I had already learned all I needed to know for my spiritual evolution, right?

I heard Katie's voice in my head, asking "Who would you be without needing to know the reason?" The truth is, there is absolutely no way to know 100% for sure *how* I got cancer. There are endless theories that can lead to a painful obsession of seeing everything as causing cancer. It was actually terrifying to look at life this way. I also noticed that blaming myself—"*I created my cancer, I could have prevented it.*"—didn't exactly help the situation either; it only created deep shame and a stigma around being "sick."

How is reality good? I was 34. Young. Healthy. Happy. This reality was still true, even with the new label of cancer. When I thought about it, it really was the BEST time for me to have cancer, wasn't it? I had a healthy physical vehicle, positive mindset, and the time and support to take care of this.

Thank God we had just moved back to Dallas, close to phenomenal medical care. This would have been a pain in the butt to deal with while running the B&B out in the country. I could see it…a guest complaining about their pillow and me replying with, "Oh yeah!!!??? I have cancer, you asshole!"

Career-wise, I had been about to launch into much more work, but this was not the time to add any extra clients or events to my plate. I still had a small group of private clients who had been with me for years and who would be understanding if I needed to shift things around or cancel classes as I underwent treatment. Yoga was actually an amazing job to have as a cancer patient as it could keep me active, moving, and relaxed.

I had massive support from my family, friends, and medical team, and I was soon awestruck by the indescribable benevolence and generosity of human nature.

Best of all, I had unwavering inner support. I had the tools to fall into a deep appreciation for cancer. *How do I know?* It was already happening. I knew how to take care of my mind and body through inquiry and movement, through managing the emotional and physical aspects of treatment and side effects. I also knew how to live a healthy lifestyle through eating plant-based foods and going to healing workshops and acupuncture, and I might be introduced to even more complimentary healing paths.

Wow, it really seems as if I have been training for cancer for the past ten years. As these epiphanies hit me, I realized that although I couldn't answer *how* I got cancer, I did know *why*: for self-realization.

I gently caressed my Lulus and thanked them for showing up. "You really are my little Buddhas, aren't you?"

At around 6:00 pm, I realized that my head was pounding and I hadn't eaten lunch. Travis jumped up to prepare dinner for me. He said, "You don't have to do anything around the house anymore, honey. I'll do all the cooking and all of the cleaning. I'll go get your car washed too. I'll work. I'll take care of everything." *How thoughtful!* (And how incredibly unrealistic.) We had no clue just how rocked our marriage was about to be. But for this moment, I was more than happy to be on the receiving end.

My dad sent me a text saying how proud he was of me for how I was handling this. I agreed. I was pretty damn proud of myself that day. We proceeded to text hilarious emojis back and forth… my favorite being the poop emoji with big eyes and a smiley face. (No, it's not chocolate ice cream, people.)

The breast surgeon called, sharing that she could make time in her schedule for the consultation in two days so that we could begin further diagnostic testing right when my insurance kicked in. She even offered to comp the visit since my insurance wouldn't be active yet. *Wow. Kind. Universe.*

I cleared my work schedule for the rest of the week, feeling like my healing team and plans were all coming together.

Around 8:30 pm, my body and mind just fully let go. I crumpled into child's pose onto my purple yoga mat sprawled over the hardwood floor of our living room, and the tears began a-rockin'. Deep wailing, shaking, moaning…I just let it all out. At one point, I found myself hovered over the toilet, dry heaving. To an outsider, I probably looked like someone who was deeply suffering.

But that wasn't my experience.

It wasn't painful. It felt like the body needed to go ahead and do its thing. Luckily, I had had enough experience with emotional processing to know that all I needed to do was get out of the way. I'm not sure how long this went on. Eventually, I ended up in bed with Travis massaging my head, drifting off, emptied, and at peace.

September 16th—the day of my diagnosis—officially became my Cancerversary. It's a day I fully celebrate. It's the day my life took a beautiful new direction. Perhaps "New Direction Day" is a better name for it.

I suggest that you not do The Work with the motive of healing your body. Go in for the love of truth. Heal your mind. Meet your concepts with understanding. I love to say that when you finally get your body totally healthy, it may get hit by a truck. So can we be happy right here, not tomorrow, not in ten minutes— can we be happy right now? I use the word happy to mean in a natural state of peace and clarity, and that's what The Work gives us.

—BYRON KATIE

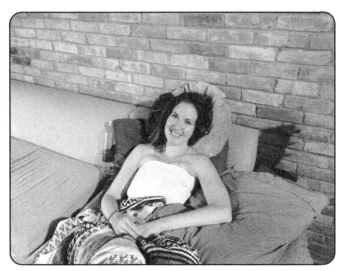

Biopsy Day

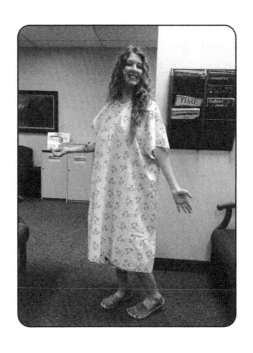

5 STEPS TO CLEAR SCANXIETY

1. **Connect with your breath.**
   Notice where your breath is in your body. Begin to focus your breath on your belly. Take a deep breath in through the nose, then a nice long exhale out through the mouth.

2. **Touch something solid.**
   Use your hands to touch something solid—the chair, a wall, the table. Feel the floor beneath your feet, your hips on the chair, or your back or stomach on the exam table.

3. **Notice your surroundings.**
   Become a witness of what is around you. See the shapes, colors, and textures. Notice the sounds: the voices, the music, the machinery. Take in the smells (ok, maybe not!). Observe the movement of people around you. See the kindness in people's eyes.

4. **Question your thinking.**
   If you feel stress, pause and notice your thoughts. If you notice you're thinking about a scary future, *This will be painful...The results will be bad,* ask yourself these two questions from The Work of Byron Katie: *Can I absolutely know it's true in this moment? Who would I be without the thought?*

5. **Remember it's all here FOR you.**
   The doctors, the nurses, the staff, the paperwork, the needles, the drugs, the lighting, the equipment, the music, the warm blanket...it's all here for you. To support you. To get a clear picture of what's going on in your body. To help you heal. To show you the next step.

5

Why I Don't Fight Cancer

IT WAS MY FIRST DAY WITH CANCER...*Oh wait, I guess I have had it for years already.* Correction: this was the first day that I was *aware* of having cancer. I had the morning to myself, and, surprisingly, it was pretty magical. First, my morning "steam & tizzle." This was a new ritual for me involving boiling chopped ginger and turmeric root in purified water, placing my face over the steam and breathing it in for a few minutes. It cleared my head and felt like a mini-facial. I then would drink the tea with homemade organic nut milk and raw honey—it tasted incredible on top of its natural anti-inflammatory, immunity-boosting, and anti-cancerous properties. *Boom. I'm so already rocking this cancer thang.*

During my morning walk through Reverchon Park, I felt so present, like the best high I'd ever experienced—the vibrant shapes and colors, the way the sunlight streamed through the trees, casting dancing shadows over the pavement. A gentle breeze brushed my face, signaling that the hot-ass Texas summer was finally coming to an end. The sound of birds chirping, traffic zooming…it was all just so beautiful. *I'm baffled—has it always been like this?* There was this lively sense of quiet calmness inside of me. *Life is simple. Life is beautiful. Wow.*

At the end of the walk, I stopped and chatted with the property manager at our condo complex. He said, "I don't mean to pry, but you're in such great shape and you're so beautiful—do you really just do yoga? I mean, you look like you're in your twenties." He had just had a phone consultation with my wellness coach husband last week, getting tips on food, exercise, and stress relief.

"Yes, it's mainly yoga, walking, and I do love rebounding and swimming. Healthy foods are important to me, and I've learned to listen to my body and eat what feels good—I've been known to rock pizza and a turkey burger too. I also think the most important thing is to take care of the mind. We use The Work of Byron Katie to deal with stress. When the mind is stressed, the body's systems don't work as efficiently."

I felt myself begin to turn "sharing my experience" into being all teachy and shit. So I blurted out, "But crap, what do I know—I just found out yesterday that I have cancer. So yes, you can do all of these amazing things for your body and mind…and still get cancer!"

God it feels good to be blunt and honest. I mean, really, what do I know about health for anyone else? Living this way felt right for me: natural, kind, nurturing. I wanted to continue to live this way to support healing from cancer.

I would later learn that freaking out, throwing parties, bargaining with God while in intense pain, and having emotional exorcisms would also be part of my healing path…but now I'm getting ahead of myself.

In the afternoon, I picked my mom up from the airport. *My*

mommy is here! My mommy is here! I was transported back to grade school as I jumped out of the car and zoomed in for one of the BEST hugs I've ever experienced. There is always something so soothing and comforting about being nestled into my mother's chest. *I. Am. So. Happy. She. Is. Here.*

The next morning, completely out of character, I woke up at 5:30 am and spent a quiet morning in the dark with my mom sipping organic decaf jasmine tea and doing some gentle yoga. In the midst of hamstring stretching and hip opening, the tears started up again. Mom placed her hand on my back while I was in pigeon pose and stroked my spine. I love her so much and felt so close to her that morning. I fell into her arms as we cried together.

My very first yoga class was led by my mom when I was 15. It was an awesome way to de-stress from my over-achieving-perfectionist high schooler's mind. I actually fell asleep at the end of every class; she often needed to give me a little wake-up nudge because I was snoring. Some yoga teachers consider it an insult for students to fall asleep at the end of a yoga practice. I see it as the ultimate compliment.

Mom and I had a great relationship while I was growing up. After all, we were the only girls in our family of five. However, we went through rockier times in my twenties. My rebellious phase came later in life, and she became an easy target for me to blame all of my problems on. It was that phase of growing up when you realize that your parents aren't God but mere mortals. They have emotions, belief systems, and are influenced by their own past experiences. So obviously, if there was a flaw in my personality (i.e., difficulty speaking my truth or issues dealing with anger), it was their fault.

My parents weren't 100% on board with Travis at first, and now that I reflect on it, I can't blame them. The timing of meeting him coincided with so many personal changes in my life, and I had begun to pull away from them. Travis represented a more non-traditional, idealistic way of thinking and living, one in which the priority was to "follow your heart no matter how crazy it sounds." On top of that, we were engaged only eight months after meeting each other, and over half of that time was spent with us living in separate countries. Naturally, any parent would view him through the lenses of over-protective sunglasses. While I have no doubt my parents wanted me to be happy, I also had the impression that, for them, a more traditional life with steady salaried jobs and five- or ten-year plans would give them a sense of security, of knowing their children would be OK.

I must clarify that I wasn't the only rebel in the family. All three of us kids have given them quite a run for their money! My younger brother, Jordan, was a chef who biked across America after college and had recently returned from traveling around the world with his fiancée. My older brother, Ryan, and his wife were devout members of an ashram in Florida, and Ryan was a firemedic who would soon begin a new career in Chinese medicine.

So yeah, nothing traditional going on here. And I love that about my family.

But dear God, did I go to war with my parents to fight for my new spiritual, hippy-dippy life with Travis. Shit hit the fan after our Moon Wedding. "*Wait—what wedding?" you ask*?

Yes, our Moon Wedding—not to be confused with our Wedding Retreat at Living Waters. This was our first wedding. We had been engaged for two years, and I had no motivation to plan any type of ceremony, but I was also sick and tired of calling him my fiancé and hearing people ask, "So when's the big date?" A wedding felt so typical, so conventional, like too much unnecessary work and a waste of money. Plus, why do you need a piece of paper to say you're husband and wife?

So on New Year's Eve, we decided to secretly marry ourselves. I bought a wedding dress, we got our fav foods from our fav restaurants, and sipped champagne. Under a full moon at Turtle Creek, we exchanged our vows. It was spontaneous, crazy romantic, and so intimate.

Turns out my parents didn't see it as crazy romantic—they just saw it as crazy. They were angry, hurt, and outright refused to acknowledge our marriage as "real" without a legal certificate. When I told them we still wanted to have a wedding party to celebrate with friends and family, my dad said he wouldn't attend. I felt devastated, rejected, and full of rage. *Why couldn't they just accept my new life? Why was their love conditional?*

My war with my parents sent me and Travis to a Byron Katie workshop in Houston. I had just read Katie's book, *I Need Your Love, Is it True?*, which focuses on how to stop seeking love, approval, and appreciation from other people and to find these things within yourself instead.

My heart was racing as I raised my hand to speak in front of an audience of 700 people. Public speaking absolutely terrified me, but my desire to overcome this pain about my parents left me no choice. I stood up, wrapped a shaking hand around the microphone given to me, and shared with her my appreciation for this book that sounded like the story of my life. Standing on the stage, Katie wore a warm, welcoming smile, and the big screen behind her revealed her serene blue eyes. I then explained the situation with my parents to her and the crowd of strangers.

She invited me to role-play with her, assigning me the role of my parents and her speaking as a more clear-minded me. Her instructions? To come at her with every painful criticism that had ever come out of my parents' mouths. I'll admit, it was kinda fun—I got completely lost in the role as I raised my voice, called her crazy and woo-woo, proclaimed that she would never be married in the eyes of the Catholic Church (even though my parents aren't religious). I accused her of just drinking her husband's Kool-Aid, dismissing all this "speaking your own truth" as mystical bullshit. The audience roared with laughter. But Katie? She received my rage with a calm, compassionate understanding. She nodded her head in silence. She didn't defend or justify herself. When I had run dry of accusations, a crisp silence filled the auditorium.

She looked me directly in the eyes and said, "Awww, honey, they miss you."

This truth nearly knocked me over; it hit me right in the heart. Tears welled up in my eyes and I began to sob. "I miss them too." So. Much.

I flashed back to one of our recent arguments in which my dad had said, "We miss the old Beth." While that hurt like hell in the moment, I could now take in his words with an open mind. I realized that I, too, missed The Old Beth. The Old Beth who got along with her parents. The Old Beth who didn't need to be "right" all the time, the one who could just go with the flow, be happy, and have fun with anyone.

Katie's words came to mind. "Would you rather be right or happy?" *BOTH DAMMIT! OK, fine…I'll take happy, please.*

The truth is, my parents weren't the only ones uncomfortable with the new me. I was still getting to know myself and wasn't always cozy in my new skin. If I was no longer the hard-working, partying, social butterfly, then who was I? I became conscious of an internal unease, an internal war, and I was projecting it out onto them. *If I'm not loving myself unconditionally, how can I expect others to do it?* With my newfound clarity, I saw how they were just like me—we were all finding our way through a fog of confusing emotions and beliefs.

The drastic shift in awareness I experienced in that weekend workshop motivated me and Travis to attend Katie's nine-day *School for The Work* in Los Angeles as our "honeymoon." Predictably, my parents weren't on board with this decision either, since they had found some online article labeling The Work as a cult. Yet I knew it was the right decision for us.

Through inquiry, I discovered that the root of my stress and suffering had nothing to do with my parents. I became aware of the super-obvious reality that I lived in Dallas and they lived in Florida but would still get so pissed off and frustrated about them on a daily basis. They weren't even physically near me, so how could *they* be the source of my problems? I began to see that the problem really lay in my thinking about them. They lived in my head! In my mind, I'd rehash our past arguments, defending and justifying my life over and over again. Were those my real parents in my head or were they images?

It dawned on me: they weren't real. I was reacting to images, to pure imagination. That's when I suffered the most.

Inquiry allowed me to revisit those past arguments and re-experience them with a clearer mind, especially during Question 4: *Who would I be without my story of them?* I was able to see how much my parents loved me and wanted the best for me. Now I could hear their feedback and ideas about how I should live my life without taking it so personally. Instead, I could hear it as love.

I could also see that a huge reason they were so upset about the Moon Wedding was that they had wanted to be with me for that magical day. That's a day parents dream about for their children, especially their only daughter. How did I not see this before? And ya know what? I so wanted this too.

Two years later, my dad walked me down the stone aisle of our Wedding Retreat at Living Waters. At last, we got to have our father-daughter dance, and he performed his infamous Magic Show at the reception. (Think grown man setting all pride aside, humming the tune of a circus clown, and performing magic tricks that a three-year-old could accomplish. It's. So. AWESOME!)

Less flashy, but still endearing, my mom read a touching poem at the rehearsal dinner, and we had our hair, nails, and makeup done together. The last day of our Wedding Retreat happened to fall on Mother's Day. All of the children and spouses surprised the moms with a cake and heartfelt speeches about how much we loved and appreciated them. There wasn't a dry eye in the room.

My relationship with my parents has evolved and deepened so much over the years, likely due to the fact I stopped being such an asshole to them. At this point, we are now so close. I'm beyond grateful. And all it took was an inner shift of perspective—the willingness to see love in all things. The willingness to drop the war, drop the fight, and use the challenges as a path to self-realization and self-growth. A perspective that turned out to be the foundation for my approach to cancer.

Fighting cancer doesn't work for me. (And it's completely OK if it works for you!). For me, when I go into fight mode, I'm closed, hardened, and operating under an illusion of false power. I feel the armor on a physical level. It shuts down my breath, my shoulders climb up to my ears, my body is literally in a fight-or-flight stress response mode. I become blind to how a challenge is serving me. It hurts. When I drop the fight and truly accept I am meant to be on this journey, that's when I feel real power. A calm. An openness. An inspiring sense of resilience. Why would I fight when I could be this free instead?

When I hear cancer referred to as a battle, it signifies that there is a winner and a loser. That's a lot of pressure! Every person facing cancer is a winner regardless of the outcome. It takes an immense amount of courage and strength to even just wake up in the morning after hearing those three life-changing you-have-cancer words. Again, if going to battle helps you to feel empowered, by all means fight your fight! I just want to share that I found another way that really worked for me. Fighting was just never required in my experience. Instead, I chose to welcome my guru.

Back to my parents. I was just over-the-moon grateful that Mom could be here in Dallas and share this journey with me. Just a few months ago, we were leading our first Yoga & Meditation Retreat together in the monkey-filled jungles of Costa Rica, a trip that completely solidified our newly discovered bond. *Perfect timing.* Not only did I appreciate her love and support in being with me, she was also a registered nurse. Her medical mind and expert caretaking skills became invaluable during this process as I learned an entirely new language, a new world that was completely foreign to me. *I mean, what's an oncologist again?*

The world will be at war for as long as the mind is at war with itself. If we can't find peace within ourselves, where is the hope for peace in the world?

—BYRON KATIE

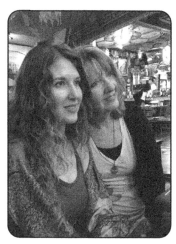

Mommy and Me in Dallas

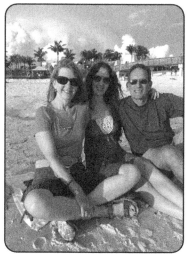

My Parents in Fort Myers

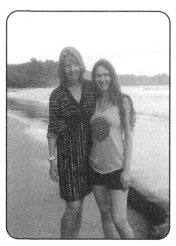

Costa Rica

6

The Treatment Plan

I WAS ALL DRESSED UP, which for me meant not wearing yoga pants, for my first appointment with the breast surgeon. I decided to wear super-sexy underwear, telling myself that if things got stressful, I could always remind myself that I was wearing a secret, doctor-not-approved baby pink thong…hopefully bringing some comic relief to a potentially crappy situation.

While sitting between Mom and Travis in the waiting room, I met my Health Navigator, who handed me a massive binder of information on everything from cancer education to treatment procedures to tips for health and wellness. I was so excited to see recommendations for writing, yoga, acupuncture, healthy diet, humor—this was my wheelhouse! The Health Navigator told me she was here to support me through the entire process and that their team cared about my wellness as a whole. According to her, they wanted to hear from me anytime. I now had the cell phone numbers of everyone on the team along with a promise that they would always return my call the same day. I was starting to become impressed with Western medicine. It wasn't the cold, impersonal, big pharma-driven industry I had imagined.

This was obviously the opportune time to take a "cancer selfie" in the waiting room. My first cancer photo…but wait, I had unknowingly been taking cancer photos for years now. I had to admit that so far I looked pretty damn good with cancer. And even more confusing, but good news, I *felt* really damn good with cancer. Aside from the whirlwind of believing stressful thoughts as if they were some kind of addictive candy, I was surprisingly calm in the waiting room.

Wearing a big smile, I met the breast surgeon in the exam room. When she asked, "How are you doing?" I responded, "Well, I'm extremely happy to see YOU!" Surprised by my reaction, she commented that she was usually the last person patients wanted to see. I didn't understand why. I mean, she was the cancer expert lady, and isn't that who you would want to see ASAP if you have cancer? So much better than consulting Dr. Google.

As she conducted a manual breast exam, I pretended to ignore the extremely worried look that crept over her face. She took measurements of my Lulus: the large lump in my breast, the lump in my armpit, plus the NEW breast lump that I had discovered the night before.

After I got dressed, we all gathered in her office. At Mom's insistence, I recorded the conversation so that we could use it for reference later if needed (P.S. This is a BRILLIANT idea for ALL medical appointments—your memory gets mushy as shit super quick!).

I assumed the treatment plan would be pretty simple: we would talk about a small surgery and then maybe a little chemo… I'd be cancer-free by the end of the year, no biggie.

Apparently, I was very naïve.

She launched into the chat by telling us that the cancer was extremely aggressive, which is common in younger bodies.

Gulp. Think of the sexy underwear…think of the sexy underwear…ugh, it's NOT working.

She went on to report that there was a large tumor in my breast, about 4.2 cm, and it had spread to my lymphatic system, meaning cancer was definitely traveling throughout my body. We didn't know how many lymph nodes were affected, but the largest lymph node tumor was about 4.8 cm.

She pulled up a screen to illustrate how the cancer cells form in the breast ducts and then multiply and divide, but it was all one big blur to me. *Aggressive? Really?* I explained to her that I wanted to keep my breasts and would want to opt for a lumpectomy. Losing my fantastic boobs was absolutely not an option for me. To my dismay, she told me that the masses had grown too big for surgery at this point, especially in the armpit. If she were to do surgery, it would be mutilating to my body and could result in possible nerve damage or the loss of the use of my left arm. OK, I'm pretty fond of my left arm, so I reluctantly agreed that it sounded like a good recommendation.

She didn't think that the cancer had taken root anywhere else yet, although a series of diagnostic tests would be ordered for the day my insurance would take effect just to be safe.

Wait…there's actually a chance it's terminal?

She then recommended kicking off the treatment plan with neo-adjunctive chemotherapy, which would consist of an initial five to six months of chemo with the goal of shrinking the tumors and mopping up any remaining cancer cells that may have spread throughout my body. Surgery would follow the chemo, and hopefully the shrinkage could make me a candidate for a lumpectomy.

Then six weeks of radiation. Then ten years of hormone therapy.

Shit. That was wayyyyy more than I was expecting.

It's a very odd sensation to hear someone tell you things about your body and not be able to feel any of it AT ALL. *Then again, would I want to feel this?* Maybe reality is kind in this way. It makes it so surreal though. *Is she really talking about MY body? I have cancer AND it's this serious, really?* On a positive note, she mentioned that the survival rate is really good for this type of cancer: 85% after treatment.

Wait a minute…there's a SURVIVAL rate? Is there really a chance of me dying? All my mind could focus on was 15% death, and that 15% felt like 150%. *I could die of cancer in my thirties. WTF.*

My mind started a slideshow of pictures of Travis with his second wife after the first love of his life died of cancer. This thought was unbearable. She was gorgeous, by the way, very exotic looking with long dark hair and deep green eyes…she was a wonderful mother to their children, and he was happy with her. I would become just a fading memory.

Yet, here I was. Alive. In the office. Still married.

I told the doctor how confusing it was to hear this information because I felt so healthy. I had thought I would be able to know something was off. Geez, I had built a career out of being "in tune" with my body. I guess I wasn't as intuitive as I thought.

She looked me right in the eyes, saying, "You feel healthy because you are healthy." *OK, I think I like her.*

I asked in a shaky voice, "Will I lose my hair?"

"Yes. Within the first few weeks of chemo."

Ouch. That stung. My hair. My boobs. My two favorite parts of my body. I was known for these things! Don't you know I'm the girl with the mermaid hair, double D boobs, and a size two yogini bod? That's ME dammit, and this "me" was being threatened on all levels. In high school, I had the nickname "PT", which stood for "Perfect Tits." In fact, some guys actually created a chant for them: "Beth's breasts are the best!" *Sigh.*

The surgeon wrapped up our meeting by saying she would set up an appointment with the oncologist right away and schedule the tests. *Oncologist?* As we said our goodbyes, I started to feel my body tremble. I was barely holding it together.

As we walked out of the office door, I completely fell apart. My legs stopped working. Travis held me up as we stumbled through the lobby and parking lot. Mom grabbed the keys and instructed us to sit in the back seat together. Exhausted, I collapsed into the car and began wailing in his arms.

There was no stopping my mind from going all over the fucking place. Fear of death, pain, suffering, consumed me. *This wasn't part of my life plan!* Anger, confusion, terror, shame, panic. *This shouldn't be happening to me. The cancer is spreading. I will die young. My body betrayed me. Treatment is poisonous to my body. Chemo will make me look sick and ugly. The side effects will be unbearable. I should have gone to the doctor sooner. I can't handle this. My life is over!*

Yet what was reality in this moment? Girl in the car, being held by husband, mom driving. Although it was one of the hardest moments…although this part really sucked ass, I was still in touch with the support and kindness of reality.

Once I was home and the tantrum passed, I revisited this stressful moment in the car and wrote down the mind-vomit list of stressful thoughts. As I met each thought with inquiry, I gathered more and more proof that suffering only existed in my mind. It was what I was *imagining* that might happen that created my stress. It was what I was *believing* about cancer, about chemo, about my future that sent me down the rabbit hole. What's more, what I was believing wasn't even real in the moment. It was a movie!

Granted, it was a scary one. But in reality, I was in the car, being held and driven home, and this reality really was kinder than the movies playing in my head. I wondered if this truth would hold throughout treatment and committed to continue testing it.

What was most alive in my head at that moment was the belief that *the cancer is spreading*. It had popped up multiple times: when I found a new, third lump in my breast, when the breast surgeon told me the cancer was "traveling," when I felt intense pain in the back of my neck, and when I got a migraine. All of these situations unfolded the same way: I felt or heard something, and that thing meant…*the cancer is spreading*.

It can be helpful in inquiry to focus on one situation—one moment in time—when we believed the thought. In this case, I chose to meditate on the night before my appointment with the breast surgeon. I was at home, sitting on the couch in the living room. Mom and Travis were nearby. I was exploring my left breast with my fingers and felt a new lump. The thought hit: *the cancer is spreading*.

Is it true? Yes.

Can you absolutely know that it's true? No.

How do you react, what happens, when you believe the thought that the cancer is spreading? I felt the lump and a huge wave of panic came over me. My heart raced, breath shortened. I sensed a constriction in my heart and my throat, and I slouched forward to protect myself. I frantically began to press on the lump and the area around it, convincing myself it was a new tumor. Immediately, I had an image of the future, one in which the tumors continued to spread throughout my entire body at a rapid rate. I saw cancer taking over my organs, my life, my happiness. I saw an early, sad, painful death. I felt helpless, hopeless, out of control, and absolutely terrified watching these images. I treated myself like a victim, and then I started to bully myself for not getting the first lump checked out earlier. *I could have prevented all of this; it's my fault.*

I asked Mom to feel the lump, and I studied her face. *If she looks panicked, then I will panic even more.* She seemed calm, but I suspected she might have been putting on a show so I didn't freak out. I couldn't listen to Mom or Travis as they tried to comfort me. *They don't know what it's like.* I'm angry and confused at my body—*how could you do this to me?* Then I turned on God—*what the fuck kind of lesson are you trying to teach me here, asshole?* I didn't want to deal with this, and at the same time, I felt an immense pressure and sense of urgency to do something quickly before my body became one big tumor.

Who would you be without the thought? I noticed my surroundings and that I was sitting in the living room. *It's quiet, I'm comfortable on the couch.* I felt the lump and I was curious. Without the label *the cancer is spreading*, the lump was simply *interesting.* My mind was more open and calm, allowing me to see many possibilities: *maybe it's inflammation, a cyst, swollen lymph node, who knows?* I added the newest Lulu to my list of questions for the next day's appointment with the doctor. I was able to be present, not focused on the future. Even when I did, the future looked simpler. I was at ease taking things one step at a time. *Right now, relax on the couch with my family. Tomorrow, go to the doctor. Ask questions. Await next steps.* Without the thought *the cancer is spreading*, I was free to show the lump to mom and hubby without a dependent need for validation from them. I loved having them both there with me and felt supported and connected to them, to me. My body relaxed, breath deepened, throat softened. I appreciated my body showing me the lump so I could learn more. I didn't give the lump a label either, didn't rate it as bad or good or cancerous or benign—it just was. In fact, there was even a hint of excitement about launching into this brand-new journey into the unknown. I became much more relaxed and at peace.

When I turned the original thought *the cancer is spreading* to its opposite, it became *the cancer is not spreading.* What are some examples of how this could be true? *It could be inflammation—I did have a large biopsy needle and anesthesia needles poking into my breast multiple times only a few days ago. It might be a swollen lymph node or a cyst like I've had in the past; I know my body is good at making them! I have absolutely no proof or solid evidence that I am feeling a cancerous tumor. It's just a story I made up about a lump. I mean really, where is my proof? I can't actually see cancer cells. I can't even feel cancer—I simply feel skin, something hard and bumpy.*

I then turned the thought around to my thinking: *the cancer in my thinking is spreading. Holy crap, this is even truer—right now, the only place the cancer is definitely spreading is in my mind.* In my imagination, my entire body was full of tumors that would continue to take over until my painful death. I asked myself, "Is that real or an image?" *It's total BS (belief systems). The reality is that I'm on the couch, very much alive, feeling a lump. It's the story I put on the lump that is creating my suffering and panic. Not cancer. These scary stories are multiplying one after the other, just like cancer cells divide and spread. Geez, they're more painful than cancer!*

I also turned the thought around to the other: *I am spreading the cancer.* How might this also be true? Well, when I believed the stressful thought, *the cancer is spreading*, my body reacted. It panicked, my heart raced, I caved forward, I was in fight-or-flight mode. This could upset the body's natural healing process. So even though I could see my innocence in going along with this thought, I could also see that if I didn't intercept thoughts like this with inquiry, I would be creating quite a hostile environment in my body, possibly even an environment where cancer could spread more easily. This turnaround helped me feel empowered, as if I was part of the healing process. Another example of how *I spread the cancer* was by freaking out to my mother and husband by showing them the lump and labeling it as "cancer spreading." *I'm having a meltdown— everybody else needs to join my panic party please!*

Sometimes the Yahoo! Turnaround is available. This is a way to look at the original stressful thought and add an exclamation point to the end of it. *The cancer is spreading! Yahoo!* This turnaround is a way to ask: *Assuming it is true, how could this be good? How could this serve you?*

I was surprised to find a whole pile of examples. *If it has spread further in my breast, it hasn't spread very far from its original source. Doctors already have a recommended treatment plan, which gives me a direction for what to do. I can notice that even if it's spreading, I'm still OK in this moment. In fact, without my stressful thoughts, I feel at peace. Happy. Healthy. Sitting on the couch. If cancer continues to spread, I would literally be forced to live in the present moment. Which could be...awesome. The bullshit things that used to annoy me (my husband being late, dirty dishes in the sink, my mom worrying too much) might melt away. What's important is life, together, now, and I don't want to waste another moment not appreciating everything and everyone in it.*

Yahoo! The cancer is spreading! I had trained for this. I was able to identify what I was believing about the cancer spreading: *I won't live a happy life. Cancer will kill me. My life is over.* Thoughts like this could be taken to inquiry, and I could already see they were complete BS. I felt motivated to clean up my lifestyle even more... it was actually exciting. Healthier foods, daily yoga, acupuncture, rest, nature, more inquiry, travel when possible...all with the intention of healing. Living life in my own private retreat sounded pretty nice, actually.

Cancer has a right to live. How do I know? Because cancer cells were living in my body. That was reality. And I wasn't in charge of when they left. But I could do my part by getting the best doctors, showing up for treatment, and taking care of my body, thoughts, and emotions. Whether it lived or died was not my responsibility—that responsibility rested in the hands of the doctors, medicine, and the universe. I could take care of the cancer in my mind, right there and then, using inquiry, so I could actually live in peace whether or not the cancer spread. *Wow.*

The irony of this situation was that the lump disappeared before the day of my additional diagnostic testing with the breast MRI and CT scan. I still have no clue what it was, I'll never know for sure, but it was a gift. It provided me with a beautiful foundation for noticing the power of the mind in this process. I was sure this thought would reemerge several times throughout the cancer journey and even after treatment ended. *Unless I'm dead. Is it too early to dish out death jokes?*

I walked into the oncologist's office with Travis, Mom, and Dad. A 12' x 12' windowless, chilly room where we would soon hear the results of the recent scans. Where we would learn if it was true that the cancer had spread. A nervous anticipation filled the air. I climbed up onto the exam table, placing my bum on the freshly drawn crinkly white exam paper. Legs swinging back and forth, I distracted myself by looking up that night's movie times on my iPhone. *Hmmm….tonight will I be watching a movie or wallowing in terror because I only have two more months to live? Ahhhh, the adrenaline might kill me first!*

My oncologist flew through the door in superhero style, proclaiming, "Good news—the cancer has not spread to anywhere else in the body. It is likely an advanced Stage II or an early III." *Jes-us.* There was an audible sigh of relief from everyone in the room. I watched our bodies literally drop a couple of inches as we collapsed back into our seats. We looked at each other, tears shining in our eyes. I will always remember this very special moment. (Obviously, another selfie was in order.)

Some people do not get to hear this news, to feel this relief. I am very well aware that someday I may hear that the cancer is terminal and I have only a short time left in this world. As excruciatingly difficult as hearing that news may be, I am willing to do the inner work necessary to eventually make peace with it. (That is, after the last act of my shit show of well-deserved emotional freakouts.) In fact, I have already started this process by questioning my terrifying stories about terminal cancer and death.

Can you imagine how freely you would live if you no longer feared death? I want a fearless life. If you're ready to see this work in action, jump to the last chapter. And I invite you to then come back and read the rest of my story.

I am a lover of what is, not because I'm a spiritual person, but because it hurts when I argue with reality. We can know that reality is good just as it is, because when we argue with it, we experience tension and frustration. We don't feel natural or balanced. When we stop opposing reality, action becomes simple, fluid, kind, and fearless.

—BYRON KATIE

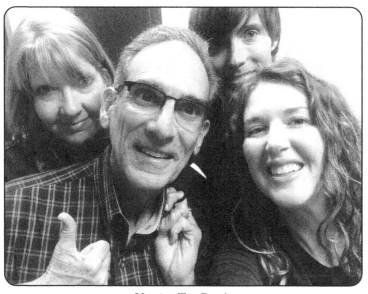

Hearing Test Results

7

Going Public &
Facing Financial Fears

TIME TO SHARE THE NEWS. *Is it weird that I'm kind of giddy?* I also wanted to be sensitive to the fact that the news of my diagnosis might be painful for some people, as they had their own frightening stories about this disease. *Wow, it actually now feels like a lie to even call it a disease.*

All of these realizations from inquiry were burning inside of me. I wanted to share my story. I wanted to share my journey in real time. I wanted to scream from the top of a mountain, "I HAVE CANCER AND I CAN ALREADY SEE IT'S THE BEST FUCKING THING THAT COULD HAVE EVER HAPPENED TO ME!"

What an unfamiliar, strange, yet arousing feeling. When it comes to sharing, I've always preferred to keep things small. I have only a few close friends. I teach private one-on-one yoga. My retreats, workshops, and teacher trainings are intimate. I spend a lot of time by myself or with my hubby. This was a new sensation: pure, raw, unfiltered inspiration. It wasn't a choice, merely a privilege to have the opportunity to articulate my experience. And social media was the perfect avenue for expressing it. After calling and emailing close friends and clients, I created a blog and a public video announcing my diagnosis and treatment plan, as well as for sharing how I was mentally and emotionally handling everything. *Who knows, maybe it will help someone. I sure as hell know writing and sharing openly is helping me.* Here's how I started:

FACEBOOK UPDATE

I have some news that may be difficult for some of you to hear. I was recently diagnosed with breast cancer. I am young, healthy, and have no family history of breast cancer, so this news came as a big surprise!

I have chosen a path of healing that integrates traditional and alternative medicine—the perfect path for me. I feel incredibly blessed to already be fully equipped with incredible healing tools—The Work of Byron Katie, Yoga, Meditation, Nutrition, Art, Acupuncture, Humor, & best of all…the Loving Support of Family & Friends.

I am not here to fight cancer. I am here to make

friends with it, listen to it, learn from it, evolve and grow. What if illness happens for our enlightenment? What if it makes our life even better? I am already learning so much from my new Guru Cancer:

People are kind.

Unconditional love does exist.

I am fully supported in every moment.

The cancer in my head (i.e., my imagination) is way worse than the cancer in reality. Whew.

The universe doesn't just pour a pile of shit on your head; there's a bigger calling at work here and I'm open to fully experiencing it. Like Byron Katie says, "Life happens for you, not to you."

You may be asking yourself, "What can I do?" There are 2 things that would really support me now:

1. Keep me smiling by sharing cute photos, funny videos, inspirational stories (especially cancer survivor stories!).

2. There is a cool daily meditation practice Travis and I are doing. Taking a few minutes

each day to imagine what it feels like for me to be completely healed. Imagine the tumors shrinking and me calling you with the news—I am cured of cancer! Feel the joy and relief, see my face...this practice has been proven to help heal illness in the self and others—can't hurt!

With Love,

—Bethany

Almost instantly, an outpouring of love and support flooded the comments section of my Facebook post. Messages from people from all areas of my life—childhood friends, old co-workers, ex-boyfriends, other cancer thrivers, friends from The Work community, from my time in Spain, distant relatives, and total strangers. There was this collective experience of oneness, of connection. Everyone was with me. It was like each person had been meticulously placed in my life by some universal intelligence to support me on this path. *I. Feel. So. Fucking. Loved.* #socialmediaspiritualityisforreal

I preferred saying, "I've been diagnosed with breast cancer" or "I'm in cancer treatment" instead of "I have cancer" because it was so much truer for me. My mind remained open to the possibility that at any moment, cancer might not exist in my body. *How can I know for sure, right here, right now? Can I touch and hold it? Spread it out over the table and show it to you?* And the insight from inquiry during the waiting game was still so alive in me—the epiphany that the majority of my body literally did not have cancer cells growing. *My toes work! My heart is pumping blood! My lungs are breathing cancer-free!*

By the way, telling people about your cancer diagnosis can elicit some really interesting, sometimes baffling, responses. Like the tendency for people to tell you how horrible this is and how their aunt's cousin's son's neighbor just died a brutal, horrific death from cancer. "I was with him until the excruciatingly painful end." *Good for you, dude.* Some would say, "Oh poor you! This is the worst! It's the toxic environment that gave you cancer! The world is coming to an end! Fuck cancer!" *That's cool, but I'm not a victim or a "fuck cancer" kind of gal.* One woman described how her breasts were dripping with blood from third-degree radiation burns. "But stay positive!" *Ummm…really?*

You also enter the land of uninvited judgment and unsolicited advice. A friend asked me, "How can you put poison in your body with chemo?" Another claimed that the only way to heal cancer was to open my heart chakra and heal my mother issues, that Western medicine would kill me. I had a friend whose relatives told her that she must have committed a sin for God to give her cancer. *Jesus, people—WTF?*

But this is part of the process for everyone going through cancer. As much as I wanted to, I couldn't control what others said. Where I was empowered—where I could and can still affect change—was by paying attention to how I reacted to their comments. At first, I'd spend a lot of my time and energy *convincing* people that I was doing great, that I wasn't suffering, and that cancer really was a gift for me. *Look at me! I'm fine! See? It's not so bad!* When they didn't seem to "get it," I'd get so frustrated. Whenever someone would offer a new suggestion for treating cancer, I'd immediately dive into a ton of defensiveness and justification for choosing Western medicine. Honestly, it was all so freaking exhausting.

I had to realize that it wasn't *my* job to change *their* story about cancer. People are going to believe what they believe. If they wanted to hear it, I could share my experience without trying to convince them or prove myself. How they responded was not my responsibility.

Additionally, I tried to remember that all of these people had good intentions. They wanted to feel a connection to me, so they mentioned a cancer story. They cared about me and wanted my body healed from cancer, so they offered advice or a book they'd heard about. I didn't have to take it so dang personally or as an implication that I was "doing it wrong." And ya know what? I realized that I also wasn't required to hang out with them! I was free to leave the conversation or not read or respond to that particular Facebook message.

I also recognized that people often don't know what to say, especially if they themselves have never been in this situation, and they may be worried they will say the wrong thing. I've been there too and sometimes still stress about it. So I am going to give you a quick and easy script for your newly diagnosed cancer friends and family: "I am so sorry to hear this. How are you doing? I'm here for you. How can I help?"

Also, be totally prepared for someone to drop off the face of the earth when they are first diagnosed—it is overwhelming on so many levels, and they may not even be aware of how people can help them. In these circumstances, you can also offer specific assistance like setting up meals for the week, driving them to appointments, taking their kids to school, hiring a maid to clean their home, or taking them on a movie date. Sometimes people simply need time and space to process what's happening, so don't take it personally if you don't hear back from them.

For the most part, I could shelter myself from the slew of scary stories and unwelcomed advice. I continued to learn to be more patient and understanding with others and myself. Still, this compassion flew right out the window when the persistent advice and judgment started coming from the person I loved and adored most: my confused husband. Travis was so not on board with Western medicine, and he was certainly not being shy about expressing it. Our cancer honeymoon phase seemed to be coming to an abrupt halt. *What's going on with him?*

While I had been diving deeper into inquiry around my diagnosis, Travis had been diving deeper into Google. While I was discovering all of the mind-blowing ways cancer could be the greatest gift of my life—how my doctors were kind and compassionate, how I felt supported by the universe, and how the nightmare was, so far, only in my head—Travis had been immersing himself in online research that claimed I was killing myself with Western medicine.

Chemo only creates cancer and kills people. Western medicine has no desire to cure cancer. Big Pharma is trying to keep you sick and profit off of you. It's all a big conspiracy (the doctors are in on it too!) and the only way to truly heal from cancer is naturally.

This was very inspiring literature to read when chemo was about to course through your wife's veins. He was having a really hard time. Yet he wouldn't question what he was reading; he believed it all and questioned my doctors instead. *Does he not remember how healthily we have lived for the past ten years and how I STILL managed to grow some rockin' cancer? Did he forget I tried working with a naturopath first whose expert advice could have killed me?* I was sure what he was reading was also true in some circumstances—there are definitely people in the world who have died because of a complication from traditional cancer treatment. And yes, there are people who cure cancer naturally too. But is this the *only* way to cure cancer? No.

Why can't we live in a world where there is more than one

"right" way to heal cancer? There's so much beauty in both sides—both are SO important and SO powerful. I think the world would be a better place if we all just got over our egos, stopped the bashing, and learned from one another. Let's face it: there are no guarantees with any path. So why don't we honor each other's choices and lift each other up? We're all doing what's right for us; we're all on a courageous path. (OK, my inspirational try-to-change-the-world rant is over. Time to come back home to my experience, my business. And honestly, I was too busy entering the next phase of my School of Cancer: The Financial Freak Out.)

Medical bills were coming in hot. The biopsy alone was now $8,000. I didn't realize that doctors could order additional tests without my permission and charge an extra $7,000 for them. Thank God I had insurance coverage for the next two months, but there was talk of eliminating Obamacare in the new year, and then what? Next year would be my most expensive cancer year: three more months of chemo, surgery, radiation, follow-up scans, and endless doctor appointments...not to mention that insurance didn't cover any of the complimentary therapies I was implementing: weekly acupuncture, Reiki, sound healing, tons of supplements, superfoods, daily juicing, and the cleanest, most organic food I could find.

We weren't Big Ballers or anything. We were essentially minimalists, and our money tended to go towards food, rent for our two-bedroom condo, Byron Katie events, travel, and private Montessori schooling for our godson. Travis and I were both self-employed and kept our finances separate. During the past eight years of our relationship, I had had a little more luck than him in the income department.

I love working. When I was 15, I started my first job as a sandwich artist at Blimpie's for $5 an hour. For some reason, as a woman, I have always felt very strongly about being financially independent. I'm capable, talented, and it feels good to support myself.

Understandably, depending on someone else financially was terrifying to me. I felt vulnerable and helpless. Not to mention undeserving. *Ohhhhh, that one stings.*

Yes, something was changing in me. There was part of me that wanted that stereotypical relationship in which a man takes care of the finances. Furthermore, since I didn't have babies at home to raise, I felt like "less of a woman" for wanting that.

Because I could work. So I felt I should work. It hit me one day that I held this belief: *I should take off work only if I'm too sick to function.* Some days I hadn't felt like working. But because I could, I did. *I don't judge others for not working, why am I so harsh on myself? What if I just take time off for no other reason than "I want to"?*

Thus, I took a break from work for the beginning of treatment. This gave me time to sort out everything—especially the medical bills—to see how my body would react to chemo, and to take care of myself. I applied for charity funds to help cover the biopsy bills and jumped on countless phone calls with medical offices and the insurance representatives to try to negotiate lower invoices and more coverage. Instead of being frustrated about "wasting my time" on these calls, I started to view it as a part-time job that would pay me if I was good at it. I stopped "wasting my time" and chose self-care during hours of on-hold classical music: rebounding, stretching, watching a show, or eating a great meal.

How else can I support myself now? By asking for what I want. I flashed back to the moment when we decided to ask the owners of

Living Waters for what we wanted: to work and live at the property. *Again, what's the worst that can happen if I ask for what I want now?* Although it was totally out of my comfort zone, I opened a GoFundMe account and asked for what I wanted, for what would bring me the most peace of mind—money.

Despite this brave step, my fearful money mind's voice grew louder and louder. The unknown was terrifying me. Travis and I sat down and did The Work together on the belief *We need more money*, and later I called The Do The Work Helpline to question the belief that *Cancer will financially ruin us.*

The ways in which I already was or could be financially supported started to come to light. This biopsy medical bill could be 100% covered by charity funds, or at least greatly reduced. We did have money in savings, not much, but enough to last for a few months. I could work a reduced schedule, which would allow time for healing and provide some financial support. During my time off, I could renew my love of making art and sell a few paintings. While I was on vacay a few years ago, I found out a big painting of mine sold, which ended up funding the trip.

I also considered focusing more on writing and turning the blog into a book. I could see the possibility of more private clients, classes, and workshops sharing The Work around pain and illness. *Wait—could it really be possible that cancer could actually financially help me and give my career a new direction?*

There was also the potential that Travis's work could grow and expand or that he would take a new job. He seemed very committed to helping me in this way. Since he was having a hard time supporting me with the medical stuff, this was the way he could contribute most. On my end, I could learn to receive and get over my egoic beliefs about being financially supported by someone else. It might even be good for our relationship.

Of course, my parents reminded me that if we were ever in a bind, they would help us. I hadn't asked my parents for money since I had started adulting, but it was comforting to know I had the option.

Without my stressful thoughts, I remembered the reality that money has *always* worked out. There have been times with more money and times when my bank account was negative, and in all of them I was always OK. *Maybe this is another universal lesson that I'm always supported? Maybe cancer is here to finally heal my financial fears.*

The Do The Work Helpline facilitator offered me a beautiful example from her own life. She and her husband had run a business together that went bankrupt. They had nothing, yet it turned out to be one of the best times in their relationship. They would curl up together in bed each night watching Katie videos. They got to see that even though they thought everything was lost, everything was actually gained. This is one of my favorite reasons for doing The Work with a partner. We always learn from each other.

Even with that lovely insight, one night all of my money thoughts came crashing down on me. There was no way in hell I could sleep—I could hardly breathe. I rolled away from Travis and began to silently weep. I'm not really a religious person; I don't pray often. But that night I was willing to try anything.

OK universe, I am really freaking out here. I need you to give me a sign that this will be OK. I raise my white flag. I surrender. Show me. And show me in an undeniable way that we are not financially fucked. (God hears more clearly if you throw in an F-bomb, right?)

The very next day, a $140 refund check from the oncology department was waiting in the mailbox. Apparently I had overpaid. I then received an email from my insurance company asking me to contact them regarding one of my claims. When I called, I learned that I had met both my deductible and my out-of-pocket maximum, meaning that everything else for the rest of the year was 100% covered by insurance. That included co-pays, medicine, tests—everything!

So…one night I surrendered and asked for a sign, and in less than 24 hours I discovered that the rest of my bills were paid for this year and the cancer people were sending me money. *Whoa.*

The blessings kept coming. My persistent phone stalking paid off, and charity covered a large chunk of the biopsy bill. The GoFundMe account collected $10,000 in donations from friends, family, and even complete strangers. Attached to each donation was an inspiring message that evoked tears of gratitude. My heart was cracking wide open.

Two girlfriends threw me a fundraiser—*could people be any kinder?* They organized a silent auction with donations from people and companies from all over Dallas: paintings, yoga sessions, cooking classes, acupuncture, handcrafted jewelry, music, and more. I had never felt so supported.

During my time off from work, Travis taught a few sessions for one of my new clients, Sophie. She loved the experience so much that she decided to continue working with him instead of me. That burned my ego, but what happened next changed our lives.

She referred him to a friend who was super well-connected in Dallas. That friend also loved Travis, so much so that she referred him out like candy and even got him featured in *Dallas Modern Luxury Magazine*. In just a few months, his client base more than doubled. *Say whaaaaat?!*

I am so grateful I had the courage to (1) admit I was struggling, (2) work my money mind, (3) ask for help, and (4) receive it when it appeared. It was an opportunity to become fully exposed, vulnerable, and surrender into the support of others and life. The kindness of others has left a permanent imprint on my heart.

Who would you be without the thought, "I need more money to be safe?" You might be a lot easier to be with. You might even begin to notice the laws of generosity; the laws of letting money go out fearlessly and come back fearlessly.

—BYRON KATIE

8

Making Friends
with Medicine

BYRON KATIE OFTEN SAYS, "If you want fear, then go get a future." I say, "If you want fear, then go read the side effects of chemo."

I plopped down at my kitchen table with a huge binder from the oncologist sprawled out in front of me. Lists of side effects assaulted my mind—hair loss, nausea, fatigue, decreased appetite, severe weight loss or gain, neuropathy, heart conditions, memory loss, mouth sores, infertility, browned fingernails, DEATH.

As I read, each word harshly hit a different part of my body. Suddenly, I doubled over with stabbing chest pains, barely able to breathe and feeling sick to my stomach. Even though chemo was still a week away, I already felt completely depleted and defeated.

But wait a minute—before I read those words, I felt fine. What happened?

Awwww crap, I had gotten myself a future. Not just any future, but a fucked future. I saw an image of future me experiencing every single side effect, not just during chemo, but for the rest of my life. In an instant, I was projecting a future of pain, suffering, and misery. My body then reacted to these images—it reacted to pure imagination—and had me experiencing the side effects of chemo before a drop of it ever entered my veins.

What's reality? Woman sitting, reading words on paper. *Holy crap-oly—the mind is powerful when you believe its BS stories.* And I kept seeing this truth over and over again: I only suffer when I leave the present moment. When I leave reality. Just look at how my body responded—believing these thoughts about side effects literally *created* physical pain, not to mention the emotional panic attack. *Could this be good news? If the mind can create pain, I wonder if it can take it away too?*

My beliefs about medicine were being deeply challenged here, not to mention the whole "natural girl" identity I had been wearing for the past decade. See, medicine and I have had a bipolar past. Sometimes I loved and appreciated it. Sometimes I feared and cursed it. These beliefs weren't new. Remember my years of intense migraines? I tried numerous alternative approaches for healing—acupuncture, massage, homeopathy, emotional clearing, various diets and cleanses, yoga therapy, meditation, sex, chiropractics, osteopathy, natural hormone therapy, and essential oils. Not to mention a few embarrassing things I tried in total desperation, like talking to a psychic and drinking my own pee. Not. Kidding.

Some of these methods occasionally brought relief (not the piss drinking…ahem, "urine therapy"), but nothing lasted. Over-the-counter medicine really did help, especially if I took it as soon as I first felt the signs of a migraine, but I still really, really resented taking it.

Then I found a six-week course with Certified Facilitators that dealt with the topic of pain and illness using The Work. The course allowed me to fully explore my thoughts around medicine, illness, doctors, physical pain, and emotional fears. My core beliefs were: *Medicine is bad for me. I want the pain to go away. I can't handle it. The pain will get worse. The pain will last forever.*

Through bringing these thoughts (and many others) to inquiry, I discovered just how much more physical pain this mental activity brought to my body. When I believed these thoughts, I was full of terror and panic; I'd start frantically searching for a "forever" cure while I was in the midst of intense pain. Naturally, my body would tense up even more—especially in my neck, jaw, forehead, and shoulders. My breath would shorten or even disappear. I would start to see myself having to cancel the rest of the activities of the day, or maybe the week…all of the things I loved to do just vanishing. I felt like a victim, and life seemed so unfair. *Someone as healthy as me shouldn't be dealing with this!* I saw images of a future lifetime of pain and agony with death as the best option. I would get easily angered by others, especially when they offered advice or tried to help. *They haven't had pain like this—they have no idea what they're talking about!* I'm sorry, but how could you NOT get a migraine believing all of this!?

Meditating on who I would be without these thoughts, I noticed that I became really curious about the first sensations I felt before a migraine hit. Pain now became a sensation. I also became aware of the story *I'm going to get a migraine,* and it was met with *Can I absolutely know it's true?* Not yet. *What's required of me now?* Through inquiry, I came to be fully available to take care of myself in the moment, which often looked like lying down in a dark room with an ice pack over my eyes, breathing, noticing, and gently relaxing any physical sensations of tightness in my body. I'd notice whether or not I would reach for medicine. And I often did. When I took it, I invited the medicine in with love and gratitude, seeing it as a healing friend. Whether it worked or didn't wasn't up to me. I was just doing my part. I focused on the present moment instead of getting caught up in what might happen in the future, becoming a witness to the thoughts and letting them float by, one by one, like clouds. *Thanks for sharing and you're not real, not real, not real.* Everything felt simpler, kinder, and honestly kind of fascinating.

The turnarounds were truer…*Medicine is good for me.* Rather than be in days of pain, which can be super stressful on the body, medicine often alleviated the pain within 20 minutes. It allowed me to spend the rest of the day doing things I loved in a body that felt calmer and more peaceful. *My thinking about medicine is bad for me.* Yes, seeing it as an enemy, especially after taking some, only created more stress and panic in my mind and body.

I don't want the pain to go away. I began to see pain as a gift, as a teacher. Actually, it was a badass yoga teacher. It helped me to slow down, get in touch with my body and breath, and take care of myself. My pain introduced me to many different forms of healing. Through pain, I've made life-long connections with others. It has helped me to become a more compassionate yoga teacher and person, giving me a reference point for intense pain. Plus, I know exactly what to do and where to touch if a client has a headache or migraine…I've been told my hands are magical. Migraines even made me better at my job!

I can handle it. Well, I can because I always have. There has been absolutely NO proof of me ever "not handling it." Now, "handling it" can take many forms: going to a doctor, taking meds, breathing, sleeping all day, freaking the F- out, crying, Netflix therapy, movement, stillness, complaining about it, it's all welcome. It's all part of handling it.

The pain will get better. Yes, it always has done this too. And at times when that hasn't been my experience, it showed me that I needed to change my approach, to go back to the doctor or try something new. I have always found that time heals, which leads to my next turnaround…

The pain will not last forever. It NEVER has. Nothing is permanent. Forever is the story of an imaginary future; it can never be real. The mind will say it over and over again, but that doesn't mean it's true. I often love to repeat the mantra *and this too shall pass.*

These realizations were monumental, and I truly began to experience pain and medicine as a gift, a privilege. It became possible to have a great life both with and without migraines because I became free to have a migraine without the suffering. Bonus: I started to get migraines less often, and when I did, they were less intense and didn't last as long. Consequently, I needed less medicine. Pretty cool side effects from doing The Work, eh?

I was clueless that my migraines were also training me for cancer treatment. Or that cancer treatment would actually end up curing my migraines. #cancerbonus

Questioning stressful thoughts about chemo and conventional treatment occupied a big chunk of my inner work at that time. I was so grateful for The Work community; countless Certified Facilitator friends were reaching out to support me in unraveling my fears. I was accepting all of their offers. The Work really was (and still is) my mental medicine. My new friend, Robyn, facilitated my journey through the game-changing inquiry: *Chemo is poisonous to my body.*

Is it true? Hell yes! I've read the list of side effects. Everybody says it, even doctors. Googling "chemo," some of the most frequent words that appear with it were "poison" and "death."

Can you absolutely know that it's true? Hmmmm, I guess I had never taken the time to meditate on if it was actually true *for me.* I couldn't 100% know for sure that it was poisonous to my body. Isn't it also healing me? My answer is, no.

How do you react, what happens, when you believe that thought? Freak out! A warning siren went off in my entire body—my stomach felt queasy, my shoulders climbed up to my ears, my jaw tightened, breath shortened. I worried I was making the wrong decision and I treated myself as an uninformed idiot playing into Big Pharma. When I believed this thought, I felt shame and embarrassment when speaking to others, especially my "all-natural" friends. I distrusted my doctors, suspecting that they didn't really want to heal me. I would take the horror stories I had heard from others, add them to the movies I'd seen, and project all that mess into a future where my quality of life was so miserable that death seemed like the only way out. In that frame of mind, I saw no possibility of joy, only worst-case scenarios. I treated chemo like something evil out to break and ruin every part of me, mind, body, and spirit. I saw my body as sick and frail, unable to "handle" the poison. I saw it seeking revenge on me by giving up and letting the cancer spread further. *I'm a terrified, lonely, hopeless victim. Wow, this really sounds like an ideal internal environment for healing cancer.*

Who would you be without the thought? This brought me back home in my body—it felt relaxed and strong. I could see how well I was doing, feeling courage, pride, and gratitude. I remembered all of the amazing women I had met who had been through chemo and were now living happy, healthy lives. Minus the thought, I was more present and positive and able to share my treatment plan with others with confidence, trusting that I was making the right decision for me. I could now see my doctors as kind, caring, and truly on my side. I remembered my oncologist's words, "I think we can cure this." I became grateful for medicine and scientific research. Chemo was a gift, a healing cleanse that was working WITH me, not against me. My job became much simpler: show up for treatment, relax, and receive. *What a relief!*

Moving on to the next part of the inquiry process, with Robyn's support, I turned the original thought around to the opposite: *Chemo is healing to my body. How could this be true?* Turns out I had no solid proof that it would poison my body. I only saw images in my mind, and they were not real. It was actually a healing cleanse that wiped the body clean of what was no longer serving it (i.e., cancer cells). *Chemo helps me to slow down and rest, so my body can focus its energy on healing.* I could still do gentle yoga, go for walks, eat, take naps, have sex, even travel. My healthy lifestyle and complimentary therapies were likely protecting my healthy cells and supporting me in dealing with side effects. *In fact, I'm motivated to be even healthier because of cancer and my treatment!* There was a lot of scientific research backing the effectiveness of chemo "therapy" (oh yeah, I forgot about the *therapy* part!).

Continuing, I turned the belief around to my thinking: *My thinking about chemo is poisonous to my body.* Examples? When I believed my stressful thoughts, my body was tense, panicked, and not breathing fully. It went into a hardened "fight-or-flight" mode, which wouldn't necessarily help the healing process. I continued to replay the stories I had heard from others in my head and gossiped about them to other people, reinforcing the "poison" image and leaving me feeling frustrated, confused, and hopeless. *I hear the poison story, I believe it. But where does the poison live right now? In my mind, not in reality.* When I went into an imaginary future of pain, suffering, side effects, and an early death, it was all just in my thinking. *Chemo itself is innocent. It's a clear or red liquid. It's my thinking about it that creates suffering in this moment.*

Turning it around to "the other" gave me: *My body is poisonous to chemo.* This one sounded weird, but I tried it on…*Ah ha!* My lymphatic system collects and moves toxins out of my body, releasing them through sweat, urine, or poooo. *My heart still beats, my digestive system works, maybe there are parts of my body, like my healthy cells, that can reject or are totally unaffected by chemo?* The reality was that my body was strong, young, and healthy.

Robyn asked, "How about the Yahoo! Turnaround?" My heart sunk a little. She was really pushing me. *Chemo is poisonous to my body! Yahoo?* How could this be *good?* She replied, "It's true because chemo is poisonous to cancer cells. Right now, cancer cells are part of your body." *Holy shit! It's true!* And the next time someone commented on how chemo is poison, I could drop the defense and agree with them. No need to fight for my perspective. I also saw how chemo being "poisonous" helped me stay really clear and consistent in my self-care practice, plus it motivated me to be creative in finding new all-natural cures for dealing with side effects.

After this inquiry, I was filled with gratitude for the gift of chemo, the gift of a healing, cleansing medicine. It deserved a new name: C-Love.

My first day of C-Love arrived during what had already been a very eventful week. Two days prior, I had undergone surgery to install my port above my right breast. I now sported a built-in plug that hooked me up to healing meds…I felt kinda like a sci-fi superhero getting her charge. It was my first big surgery, my first time going under anesthesia, so I adopted the same "wear sexy underwear" technique that had thus far proven to be 0% helpful. I have a very blurred memory of waking up in the operating room when it was over and immediately trying to sit up. As the doctors kindly invited me to lie back down, I said with conviction, "But I'm wearing sexy underwear! I'm wearing sexy underwear!" Well, at least someone got some comic relief out of it.

The day before, we had attended chemo class. The room was filled with old people with various cancers and their caregivers. The nurse guided us through every single possible way our bodies could be royally screwed by the medications, even though the chemo drugs weren't specific to our individual cancers…maybe it was some kind of liability thing to be required to take this class? Dude, if you can get out of chemo class, DO IT. Or request a private class that is tailored to your specific chemo drugs.

Luckily, I was feeling so nauseous from the anesthesia that my main focus was on not vomiting. I scouted out the nearest trashcan, drank ginger tea, and just kept breathing. I even made it through watching the old guy across from me drink bourbon-flavored Coke. Bourbon Coke in chemo class. *Who does that?*

And thank God I was in the process of learning a different way to view these crazy side effects. I used what Byron Katie calls the "don't know" mind: a mindset where I could admit the truth that I'm *not* a psychic and *can't* know the future. Trust me, when you're reading side effects, "I don't know" is where it's at. Fatigue? *Don't know.* Vomiting and diarrhea? *Don't know, don't know.* It became my new silent "don't know shit" meditation.

The nurse recommended that I take some of the anti-nausea medication, which I gladly did. Then my mind jumped into the future again, wondering if this intense nausea was going to be my life for the next six months. *Don't know, don't know, don't know.* Deep breaths.

"Is your husband OK? His face was white and he didn't look so good," a nurse asked me while we were reviewing medical coverage for the treatment. Travis had just excused himself from the room to get some fresh air. He seemed to be having a really hard time with all of this, especially the medicine. Here was a guy who hadn't taken even an aspirin for over ten years now facing the reality that his wife was about to be on massive doses of chemo and steroid cocktails.

Although he was physically there with me, I was starting to feel him pulling away. It might be more true to say that I was the one pulling away. I just couldn't be his person right then. This was all moving so quickly, and I had plenty of my own stress and my own inner work to do. I had already lined up a menu of Certified Facilitators to work with him, but he rejected each and every one, claiming that he was fine. Clearly, he was not fine. Cancer can be tough on everyone involved, not just the patient. *Why won't he just get help?*

At my mom's urging, we went for pedicures after the class. I agreed, thinking that I might feel like poo but at least my toes would look adorable for the start of treatment. The nausea meds finally kicked in, leaving me weaving in and out of consciousness during my pedicure. With a hoodie draped over my face, all I remembered was waking up with pita bread—the only thing I could eventually eat—cuddled in my arms and looking down to see my legs covered in creamy white yogurt and cucumber slices, with my pedicurist asking, "You OK, lady?" And…back to sleep.

The next day, I actually felt really good. I was ready, curious, and even oddly excited to begin C-Love. We walked into the infusion room, where I was pleasantly surprised to see a clean, bright, shiny atmosphere bustling with smiling nurses, beeping noises, and patients peacefully hooked up to IVs. This was a far cry from the dark, gloomy, screaming, murder scene my mind had imagined.

I chose a window seat overlooking trees and a small lake with a fountain. I giggled, recalling my history with fountains. In college, I had a habit of swimming in them. *Maybe one day I'll rip out my IV and take a dive into this one.*

Holy crap! This chair is so comfortable and it even has seat warmers! I began to unpack my C-Love bag filled with cancer prezzies: a warm blanket, hat, socks, adult coloring books, magazines, snacks, and mints.

While my port was "plugged in" for the first time, I held my breath to brace myself for the pain that never came. It didn't hurt. Strangely, it actually felt very secure and supportive. It was nice to know that I didn't have to be poked with needles for each infusion, since I had been told I was a "tough veiner." I usually got stabbed multiple times as nurses fished around in my insides searching for a cooperative vein. The first round of pre-med fluids began to flow, and after experiencing so much nausea the day before, I was down for any extra anti-nausea medicine…especially if the nurses called it "happy juice." *Yes, please! Bring it.*

Cozy in my warm chair, I looked around the room to scope out the other cancer patients. *Fascinating.* I didn't see pain and suffering. I saw people just living their lives. A woman and her husband sipped coffee from Styrofoam cups and read the *Dallas Morning News* together. Another woman painted her nails lavender while a man next to her nestled under a blanket for a nap. Down the aisle to my right was the cutest old guy who had paired a Superman shirt with suspenders.

Yes, I was the youngest person there by like 100 years, but I didn't mind feeling young! The woman across from me struck up a conversation with us as she applied her makeup. She could tell it was our first day. Smiling, she offered some helpful tips, like buying a great heavy-duty moisturizer and not being afraid to ask for help from others. I could see my mom's anxiety rising as our new friend told us how her mom had to move in to care for her during treatment. *Will my mom need to do the same?*

As the nurse announced that she was beginning the chemotherapy, I lay back and listened to a chemo meditation Mom had found for me. I got comfy, relaxed my body, and envisioned my healthy cells being protected and cancer cells being washed away. *Let the healing cleanse begin.*

The nurse then arrived with a syringe full of red fluid; this was the Adriamycin chemo drug often referred to as "RD" or "The Red Devil" because it is responsible for hair loss. But wasn't it truer that it was "The Red Savior"? I mean, wasn't that why we were doing this? I smiled as I watched the beautiful red liquid travel from the syringe, into the tube, and into me.

One treatment down, 15 more to go. I've got this.

Just like I made a conscious decision not to fight cancer, I made a conscious decision to make friends with medicine. After all, does your body have a better opportunity to heal when you are cursing and fearing your treatment or when accepting it with gratitude? I was determined to find the good in all things—the needles, the nurses, the drugs, even the side effects. And it was one hell of a practice!

So far, cancer treatment was showing me how to enjoy the simple pleasures of life. "Normal" everyday activities became the new awesome, especially going to Nainoa's soccer games. One day, a mother and daughter approached us on the bench, asking if anyone was in need of prayer. I replied, "Sure! I'm in cancer treatment!" (I had become accustomed to being on tons of strangers' prayer lists…couldn't hurt, right?) I assumed they would take my name, add me to their list, and move on.

Nope. Before I knew it, these women hovered over us screaming sweet baby Jesus pleas for my wholeness and safety during this tragic time. I watched in amazement at how their bodies shook, whiplashing back and forth…how their arms flailed around as they prayed for a miracle. They had no idea I was already living in a miracle. I was the weirdo who was enjoying cancer.

FACEBOOK UPDATE

Good morning…this is day 4 since my 1st chemo treatment and I'm surprising myself at how well I'm doing! In general, I have a little less energy, achy muscles, and some occasional nausea. Nothing I haven't experienced before, and I imagine this is kind of what being pregnant may feel like? What it's teaching me is to just slow down and listen to my body—lots of naps, stretching, ginger/turmeric tea, smaller/more frequent meals, meditation, walks, movies, time with loved ones. Doctors say days 3-5 can be the worst for symptoms—don't know, don't know, don't know. I'm staying present and trust that I'm capable of dealing with whatever comes up. So far, so good.

As chemo began to course through my body on a regular basis, I learned a new way to meet each unfamiliar, weird sensation. I watched the mind go into story: *I'm going to throw up! I have neuropathy! It will get worse!* My ongoing practice of inquiry automatically met the mind with *Can I absolutely know it's true?* A resounding No.

Like with the migraines, I could be fully available to myself. *What do I need right now?* Sit or lie down? Breathe? Call a doctor? Eat or drink something? Cry? Sleep? Get a snuggle? When I took the time to pause and listen, I was always led to what was needed. (I'm not trying to be woo-woo here, but test it out for yourself.)

Life was easier when I accepted that cancer treatment just wasn't a time for major "doing"; it was a time for "being." Maintaining the same pace of life wasn't possible. And this can be good news! How often have you wanted to slow down, but couldn't bring yourself to do it? Maybe you let guilt or other priorities get in the way of giving yourself this gift. Cancer and chemo gave me the green light to put ME first. And damn, I became a master in the art of napping—I'm talking morning, early afternoon, late afternoon, and early evening naps. Sometimes all in one day.

I also used my weekly chemo infusion sessions as my "me time." To be honest, I preferred to go by myself. Travis didn't seem to be capable of having fun and enjoying it with me at that point, so he mainly stuck to being my chauffeur. Through observing my husband, I could see how cancer can become an entirely different experience depending on what you're thinking and believing. Remember how I described my first day of C-Love and how all I could see was kindness, support, and people being cared for? Through that lens, the infusion room was a warm, welcoming experience.

However, Travis had walked into a completely different room. He saw suffering, unnecessary treatment, and people at the mercy of doctors and drug companies. Although standing side-by-side in reality, we were in two completely different rooms. Different mind. Different room. Perception really is everything. It was tough. I really, really wanted to change his room. I felt like he was missing out on the incredible blessings that were unfolding.

Each week, I could literally feel the tumors shrinking at a rapid rate. It was pure magic. Within two months, the 4.2cm tumor in my breast was microscopic on my CT scan, and the 4.8cm tumor in my armpit shrank to 1.2cm, giving us confidence that the therapy was also mopping up any microscopic flakes that could be circulating throughout my body.

It wasn't medicine alone that was shrinking the tumors. Around the time of my diagnosis, I had launched into eating full-on organic and vegan, drinking green juices every morning, taking curcumin supplements, and going to acupuncture every week. Daily yoga, rebounding, and walks in nature were always a priority, along with large doses of self-love and self-care. Even my oncologist noticed that the lumps were noticeably smaller before I even began C-Love. This land of combined approaches was really serving me.

I felt so much better than I thought I would. Many chemo horror stories turned out not to be true for me. I never threw up. There was never a day that I couldn't get out of bed. I did shit myself once. Now, that's just a funny story...but I'll spare you the details. Side effects were manageable with the help of ginger and turmeric for nausea, sea salt and baking soda mouth rinse for mouth sores, exercise and napping for fatigue, cold compresses and stripping in public for hot flashes, extra protein for weight loss, and fiber and psyllium husks for constipation and hemorrhoids.

At the five-month mark of treatment, I posted a video on Facebook of tiny, bald me doing a challenging yoga practice. It was titled "Is this what you thought 5 months of chemo could look like? Me neither." I am just so grateful when the mind is WRONG! And I know many bodies react differently to chemo too—so if it's excruciatingly rough for you, please, please be gentle with yourself. Please don't use my story to beat yourself up. I'm simply sharing my experience because it's what I wish I had heard when I was diagnosed.

And let me tell you, I still definitely experienced mental and emotional challenges. It wasn't all rainbows. There were some deep dives into fear and depression waiting just around the corner. But overall, C-Love had taught me that I could get through *anything*, I could even enjoy shitty times if my mind was clear and open.

Speaking of minds, I think I can read yours: *What was it like being a bald little alien for 6 months*? Oh, thanks for asking. This part of the journey deserves a chapter of its own.

I have a friend who didn't want to take medication. And I said, 'God is everything, but not medicine?' God is medicine too. So today she sees it's a privilege to take medicine. She knows that whether it's working or not is not her business. The medicine says, 'take once a day.' That's all she has to know. It's written on the bottle.

—BYRON KATIE

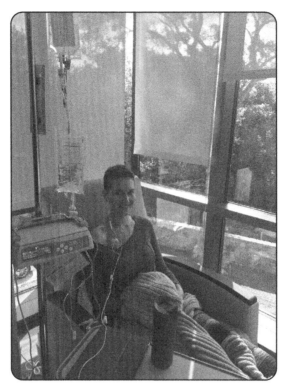

Plugged in for my 1st C-Love

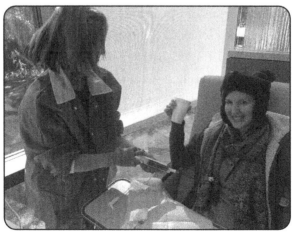

Receiving "RD" with a smile and bear hat

9

Who Would I Be Without My Hair?

I ADORED MY HAIR. By taking a hiatus from haircuts for a few too many years, my long auburn curls had finally reached official hippy "hair touching my butt" status. My hair was what made me beautiful. It was what made me feminine. The threat of losing it stirred a nauseating pain in my gut. I had never realized just how attached I was to my physical appearance; this process was waking me up to core beliefs around body image, beauty, femininity, and the fear of losing a part of "me." On top of it all, I felt ridiculous and ashamed for even caring…*it's just hair, right?*

But WHO would I be without my hair? Me. Bald. Really?

Googling "beautiful bald women," I immediately felt comforted. These women—a mixture of celebrities and regular ladies—did in fact look gorgeous, strong, feminine, and graceful.

Could bald be the new beautiful? I began to consider how easy life would be with no hair, without spending all that time on washing and styling. It took an average of 20 minutes just to comb through my hair. Sometimes it became so frustrating that I watched a short TV show on Netflix to pass the time while I raked through my rat's nest of tangles. *Oh yeah...there are things about my hair that I actually don't like!* It also cost some moolah to support this mermaid hair in the form of shampoo, conditioner, all-natural hair dye, combs, styling products, getting haircuts, hair ties...*could cancer actually save me time and money?*

It seemed a shame to let all of this hair go to waste. Someone could probably create five or six wigs from what was attached to my head. Immediately, I was struck with joy at the thought of little kids in hospitals and on playgrounds wearing my curls. If I couldn't enjoy it, why not let someone else?

Yes, this part of the cancer journey is tough...but how can I make it better? How can I support myself? How can I even make it fun?

I arrived at a decision. I would throw a hair party! A client of mine who owned a hair salon offered to open his space for us, so I created invitations reading, "Bethany's Going Back to Bald and Beautiful" complete with an adorable baldy baby photo of me. Going back to my roots. Shedding what was no longer needed. Letting go of the mermaid identity. Testing out what it meant to be beautiful and feminine.

I also wanted to remember my beautiful body exactly as it was. It would soon be changing and might never be like this again. So before my hair went bye-bye, Hubby and I set up a nakey photo shoot in our home. I was surprisingly at ease in front of the camera, taking in his artistic direction...Travis definitely seemed to be on board with this part of cancer treatment, lol. It was pretty hot! And the pictures were gorgeous. I was so happy we did this.

On a sunny Dallas Sunday afternoon, Travis and I pulled into the parking lot of my friend's salon for the hair party. "Are you sure you want to do this?" he asked. At first, I was thrown off by his question until I caught a glimpse of a vulnerable pain in his eyes…a pain that looked like it was finally ready to be seen and heard. This was about more than hair. I turned to him, "What's going on?"

My sweetheart completely broke down. Through his sobs, he gasped, "I…just…want to protect you. I thought that was my job. I just want to take it all away from you. And I can't. It's so hard for me." His weeks of inner turmoil finally had a voice, and I was finally open to hearing it. He was feeling utterly helpless. I understood that, wow, this was all really difficult for him. He was going through his own experience of what was happening to my body, and, honestly, it might have been harder than mine. Grateful he was opening up to me and admitting his struggles, I felt so connected to him in this tender moment. We held each other tight until the tears dried. "Ready to walk in?" I smiled at him as he nodded his head in agreement.

Holding hands, we headed into the salon. My family and friends all gathered around, noshing on champagne and sushi. After our toasts and a few more tears, the chopping commenced. Into the chair I went, my husband holding one hand and my mom holding the other. One friend captured the moment in video and pictures, while my future sister-in-law wrapped the chunks of auburn waves into ponytails to donate to a non-profit organization for children.

When I was twelve years old, my parents left me home alone for the first time. The mischievous me decided to freak them out by snipping off a thick strand of my blonde curls and taping it to their bedroom door. I giggled while imagining the shock on their faces, "Oh no! She's chopped off all of her hair, just like she did to her Barbies!" (Harsh childhood lesson: Barbie hair does not grow back.)

My prank has now become a family joke. Over twenty years later, my hair remained on that door. This was obviously totally normal for our family—and pretty awkward for anyone visiting my parents' home.

"I'll take over from here." Dad swooped in and snipped the very last strand of my hair as we all cheered. He later sent me a photo of it taped to their bedroom door, right next to my pre-teen strand. I burst into laughter followed by tears. *I love him.*

Walking out of the salon with my pixie cut and a new stylish dress, I felt free, alive, and even more ready for what was to come. The hair party was a way to celebrate something I knew would be difficult. Donating my curls gave me a sense of meaning and purpose, and I had now created a very special, intimate memory with my family and friends.

It was an experience I highly recommend. I've now heard of hair parties, boob parties, uterus parties, and, most recently, a "Last Supper" themed party for someone who was about to undergo a total gastrectomy (removal of the stomach due to cancer).

I am definitely pro-party! Pro-embracing challenges. Pro-celebrating things that can be difficult. Finding the silver linings.

What I didn't realize at the time was that just behind the party curtains lurked a hidden motive. I was also trying to control and manipulate what was happening to me so that I could avoid pain. *If I cut it off now, it won't be painful later.*

It was a very strange sensation living with the possibility that my hair could fall out at any moment now that I had passed the two-week mark of my C-Love experience. It was entertaining to watch my mind assume that this would occur at an extremely awkward and inconvenient time. Perhaps a chunk of hair would fall on my yoga client's face while I was giving her a massage in savasana? Or maybe it would happen in the Whole Foods check-out line...clumps of my hair appearing on the conveyor belt right next to my rosy organic apples?

The controlling me wanted to make a request of my hair: *Everything below my neck is free to go. I'm sick of shaving and don't mind a break for the next six months. Please also take my chin and mustache hair that I lovingly developed in my thirties. If you MUST take my eyebrows, eyelashes, and hair on my head...FINE...but please do it in the comfort of my own home when I have plenty of time to mentally adjust to my new Mr. Clean look. Please and thank you.*

Or perhaps I would be that anomaly who didn't lose her hair... ya know, because I'm so spiritual and all? Hey, it could happen!

It *so* didn't happen. And I handled it 100% less gracefully than I thought I would.

Around Day 16 of C-Love, I awoke at 6:00 am and just knew: *this is the day I am losing my hair.* My scalp felt tender and fragile. My fingers explored my pillow, and just like in all the stories I had read, I found a fistful of hair on my warm, white pillowcase. I got up, leaving my husband asleep in bed.

OK, this is it. I looked in the bathroom mirror and saw a still pretty hairy head. At first, I was relatively calm. I jumped in the shower because I also had read about a woman who was able to easily rub out the rest of her hair when it was wet.

Gently at first, then more vigorously, I massaged my wet scalp. Hair did start to fall out. Dark piles that looked like wet hamsters now covered the shower floor and seat. *Creepy.* The hair just kept coming. And coming. *I have so much fucking hair! How is it STILL coming out? Dear God, when will this end?* Then the water got so hot and steamy that I nearly passed out.

Stumbling out of the shower, cool air met my wet skin, and I took a deep breath. *Hey, I got this.* But then came the moment I was completely unprepared for. I looked in the mirror. A crazy lady from an insane asylum stared back at my face. *Is that ME?* Bald spots chaotically zipped across my scalp; patches of spiky, wet, thinned, old-man hair filled what was left. My look of horror paired perfectly with the rising steam enveloping me. So naturally, I did what any woman in my situation would do: I acted like a flipping crazy lady from an insane asylum.

"TRAVIS, WAKE UP! IT'S HAPPENING! MY HAIR IS FALLING OUT! GET UP! GET YOUR SHAVER!"

My hysterical screaming jarred Travis out of his slumber. "OK, honey. Calm down. But my shaver won't work for your head, it's only for faces."

"WHAT???!!!!" I frantically grabbed a pair of scissors from the kitchen and proceeded to attempt to cut off the rest of the hair that was refusing to fall out on its own. I started with the patch above my forehead, giving me an even more disturbing toilet bowl look.

Travis tried to calm me down, inviting me to breathe, put down the scissors, take a break…he promised we could shave it together later that day when he came home after work. "It can be a spiritual, bonding experience."

FUCK THAT! There was NO stopping this lady. There was only one thought on my mind and absolutely NO other options:

THIS HAIR IS COMING OUT NOW.

I ordered him to go to CVS in the pouring rain to buy a shaver. Why it took him forty minutes to get out the door was beyond me. *Can't he see I'm suffering here?!*

As soon as he returned, I charged up that baby, looked in the mirror, took in a big inhale, and G.I. Jane'd that shit off. A deep exhale left my body as I collapsed onto the toilet seat.

The best part? *It's over.* That dreaded moment was over. It became nothing more than a hilarious hairy horror story I get to tell people. You're welcome.

Later that day, I left my home without my hair for the first time. I tiptoed out the front door, looked around, inhaled deeply, and went for a walk. I stopped in a park to sit and meditate, then, leaning up against a tree, I wrote this poem:

The tree supports my spine
The hardest part is behind
Bald as can be
Feels good to be free

Of course, I also snapped my first baldie selfie and posted it on Facebook. The outpouring sea of love and support was always present on Facebook, but today it felt extra special.

The next step was showing my new look to Nainoa, which I felt a little nervous about. When he found out about my diagnosis and that the medicine would make my hair fall out, the first thing he said was, "It's going to be really weird if Bethany is bald." *Dude, I agree.*

So at the urging of my husband, I wore a scarf on my head the next morning when we met him at the Dallas Museum of Art. He was so cute. I know, eleven-year-olds aren't supposed to be cute, but I adored him. When he saw me, he said, "I heard about your hair."

I responded, "Yes, but it feels kind of cool. Do you want to feel it?"

After he nodded his head, I guided his hand to feel my smooth scalp under the scarf. "Wow, weird," he responded with curious amazement.

As soon as we got home, he asked, "SO when do *I* get to see it??!!!" *OK, I guess now is the time!* When I took the scarf off, a huge smile swept over his face. "COOL! Can we have a Nerf gun war now?" And just like that, the unnecessary nervous build-up dropped away.

I met Nainoa when he was two-and-a-half years old. Travis and I were about a month into our mind-blowing romantic escapades when he told me about a little boy he spent time with a few days a week. Travis had known him since he was born. He couldn't explain it, but he felt an instant connection to this child and somehow knew he was supposed to be in his life.

Nainoa's biological parents had issues with addiction, and, after sixteen months, it became clear they were not capable of raising him in a healthy environment. Nai went to live with his grandmother, whom he adored. Travis began to help out in little ways, like buying diapers, bringing over some groceries, and hanging out with this sweet little guy.

I wasn't surprised. Travis has such a huge heart. And as I learned more about Travis's past and how he grew up, I began to see the universe's mysterious work at play. You see, Travis's father left when he was a little boy and never came back, so he didn't grow up with a father figure around. I think meeting Nainoa sparked the heartfelt desire to give what he hadn't had.

It wasn't until I returned to Dallas after my time in Spain that

I realized just how deep their relationship ran. I distinctly remember watching Nainoa sit on Travis's shoulders in the kitchen… they were both playing and laughing. I had the thought *Wow, Travis will be such a great Dad for our kids someday.* And then the realization hit me…*wait a minute, he's already a Dad. And if he's a Dad…that means… I'm. a. mom?!* Twenty-six-year-old immature me became scared shitless at being any type of parental figure. I still had a lot of growing up to do myself! Was I supposed to be responsible for someone else? And where was the manual for a situation like this?

Luckily, I had already found the inquiry process and began to dive headfirst into questioning my stressful thoughts around motherhood. Beliefs like "Motherhood means sacrifice" and "I'm not good enough." I realized how much pressure I was putting on myself to be the super mom that *I'd* had growing up. My mom made motherhood a passionate, full-time job—she was involved in everything in our lives, from cooking all the meals to being Team Mom for basketball and president of the PTA. She could have actually gotten rid of me come kindergarten but chose instead to homeschool me until third grade. *Was I supposed to live up to this high standard?*

Doing The Work allowed me to see the reality that there were many gifts in this non-traditional, yet incredible, family situation. We got to have the experience of being in a beautiful child's life without being full-time parents. Nainoa was always cared for, and we could all have our family time, our alone time, as well as Travis and I's romantic time. I realized nobody was asking me to be like my mom except my own mind. I came to see there are *so many* different ways to be a great mother figure. This filled me with creative possibilities as motherhood transformed into a privilege instead of a requirement. It was an honor to be in this amazing child's life. I was the lucky one. Family doesn't have to come from blood. It comes from love.

I remember the exact moment I fell head over heels in love with this young boy. We had just visited my family in Florida, where Nainoa had been able to meet his new set of grandparents, aunts, uncles, and cousins. Travis, Nai, and I were the last to board the plane back to Dallas and then noticed Nai's backpack was gone. In it laid his most precious possession: Cuddle Cow. This blue-and-white striped stuffed animal with one ear that doubled as a pacifier had been in Nainoa's life since he was born. It was his security blanket, and he couldn't sleep without it. Now it was somewhere back in the restaurant in the airport terminal. *Oh crap.*

The airplane doors were closing; it was too late to grab the bag and make the flight. In a frantic state, Travis said, "Sorry buddy, looks like Cuddle Cow is gone." He continued to beat himself up about saying this afterwards, but it totally led to *my* supermom moment: I looked into Nainoa's innocent eyes and saw the tears welling up. My heart literally exploded with compassion and love for him. Then a fierce mamma bear energy—an energy I had always longed for but didn't believe I had—arose within me. "NO. I'm getting Cuddle Cow. You guys stay here, I'll catch a later flight." Nainoa's teary sweet eyes slowly looked up at me in relief and hope. Travis said, "We're coming with you," and we made quite a fun spectacle jumping off the plane together as a family on a mission. We found Cuddle Cow and spent the rest of the day cuddled up together, laughing and eating chips and salsa at the airport's On the Border Mexican Cantina. It was the best ending to our family vacation, and a new beginning of an even deeper relationship with this amazing little man. I felt beyond grateful to have him in my life. He showed me how to be silly and have fun with whatever life brings. Life is a parkour playground!

He helped me to get out of my head and into my heart. *Geez, kids are the ones who teach us.* They are the free ones enjoying life and living in the present moment.

Six years had flown by since then, and just three weeks earlier, I had found myself in the oncologist's office being asked the question, "Do you plan to have children?" Travis and I had gone back and forth many times about birthing our own baby, and we'd arrived at a "No." We both felt fulfilled as parents with Nainoa in our life. Still, a tiny part of me was a little curious as to whether we were making the right decision. Nai would make such a great big brother. "No, we don't," I responded.

The oncologist said, "Good. Because after cancer treatment, you most likely won't be able to have children, and there isn't enough time to harvest your eggs."

"Sweet! Can you guarantee that?" My reaction to her words shocked me. *Whoa. What the hell?* I actually felt *relieved* hearing this could-be-traumatic news. It's something I had been so torn about, and now it was so clear that I was not meant to be a mom in that way. I didn't have to stress over deciding anymore. And later on, years later actually, I would fully feel the grief of being infertile. The grief of never getting to be pregnant, never holding my baby in my arms for the first time, never breastfeeding. I also grieved for not being able to bond with Nainoa when he was a baby. And like all emotions, the grief eventually faded, leaving behind pure gratitude.

I marvel at how Nainoa came into my life. I was also so fortunate to have been able to hold my 3 little nieces, and one nephew as babies. Being a godmother to Nainoa and Auntie Beth to Arya, Leela, Josephine, and Rocco has been the perfect mamma medicine for me, and there are even more ways my mothering energy can be expressed. My work, the nurturing I give to my clients and the birthing of my blog-turned-book baby all allow my inner mamma to come out to play. Perhaps someday we'll get a furry baby too. I already have the perfect dog name picked out: Lulu.

I glanced over at this now sixth-grader darling boy on the couch next to me. We had rocked our family Nerf gun war and were now watching our fav show, *The Voice*. God, I really wanted to be around to see him grow up, which gave me a greater sense of purpose for healing. I adored his quick, witty sense of humor (this kid could rock some cancer jokes!), his ability to call me out on my BS, his endearing innocence, and dang, he was wise beyond his years. Out of the blue, he turned to me and said, "You know, at first I thought it would be really weird seeing you bald. But then it's like…OH! You're just the same person. Without hair!" What a little Buddha. It was as simple as that. I was still the same person. I was still me. My hair and body—no matter how they appeared—didn't define who I was.

The next night, I waltzed into Uchi, a super-trendy upscale sushi restaurant in Dallas, all dressed up and totally bald. I felt sexy, confident, and free. What a relief it was not to care what other people thought. Previously, I had worried about looks of pity or surprise or disgust. Of little children pointing and asking, "What's wrong with her, Mommy? Why does that girl look like a boy?" (Which did actually happen at a Christmas party. Little fucker. JK—I survived!)

I now realized that people don't really give a shit. They may smile and nod, but then they go on living their lives. *Wait…The whole world doesn't revolve around me?* And it's exhilarating to be *proud* of being bald. Sometimes I got high fives and hugs from strangers. Women asked if I was in treatment, then shared their victorious cancer stories. It was connecting. One afternoon, I even had a baldie lunch with my cancer friend, Amy, who was rocking the same look. At the end of our meal, the waitress informed us that a stranger had already anonymously paid for it. We both cried. *People are so kind.*

I didn't want to hide my bald head. There's this rebel in me, the one who dares to be different—she's a badass. I was almost disappointed winter was coming (WINTER IS COOOOOOM-ING!) because I would probably need to wear a warm hat. I'd been warned that you can lose a lot of body heat without hair.

I was also grateful to discover that I don't have any strange birthmarks on my scalp, like a mole in the shape of a penis or something. There was this tenacious patch of hair shaped like a crescent moon near the crown of my head that hadn't fallen out. A few cute freckles were sprinkled next to it. So I had the moon and the stars watching over me. Literally.

Surprisingly, my head is the size of a peanut. I am not kidding. Do you remember the creepy guy in *Beetlejuice* with the small head? That's me. I had no idea how tiny it was because it had always been framed by a lion's mane. What was most entertaining was that when taking group photos, we had to try to position me closer to the camera so I didn't look like a microscopic alien.

Honestly, I feel everyone should experience being bald at some point in their life. It is so freeing. You have never truly felt the breeze until it swirls over your hairless head. Everywhere I go, I now picture people bald—it's such raw beauty.

And just like the tradition of brides going wedding dress shopping, it is a rite of passage in the cancer journey to go wig shopping with girlfriends. I had no intention of buying one, but it sounded like a blast to try on different looks. I was hoping they had Afros.

Eight girlfriends—a mix from college, kickball, advertising, and yoga—all gathered one Saturday morning in front of a wig shop near Lovers and Inwood Lane. I could hardly contain myself. I tried on long wavy curls, short bobs, bangs, hot pink, even a short gray wig to mimic Byron Katie. The naturalness of the wigs surprised me. I fell in love with one in particular, a short auburn cut that parted on the side, with longer strands swooping down below my chin. I named her Samantha, and she was coming home with me.

I was going to wait to see if my insurance would cover the wig, but one of my girlfriends bought it for me (people are so kind), and we headed to my fav Tex-Mex place, Urban Taco, for lunch.

Since they were all planning to drink margaritas and I had cut out alcohol, this was obviously the perfect time to pop my first Marinol, a synthetic form of THC prescribed by my oncologist to help boost my appetite and gain weight. Yes, Texas was way behind on the whole legalizing marijuana movement. This was my oncologist's way of meeting me in the middle when I asked, "Should I smoke weed?" when hearing her concerns about my rapid weight loss. She was taken aback, "Uhhh…well, I admire your candor. Because you don't know what else is mixed in with the marijuana (true dat—one of my friends went to the ER because hers was laced with rat poison), I'd feel more comfortable with you taking synthetic THC."

Let's just say trying any kind of drug for the first time in public and on an empty stomach is…well…a dumb move. #lifelessons

After ordering our taco platters, it hit me hard. A wave of heat and panic came over me. My breath went bye-bye, and my heart felt like it was about to jump out of my chest. The restaurant got smaller. Hands shaking, I tapped my friend Jenny on the arm and asked her to sit outside with me for a moment. I then revealed that I was experiencing extreme paranoia and panic. She responded, "Oh shit! You're not going to do what you did in college? ARE YOU?"

"Shut up, Jenny. Just. Be. Calm. And. Pet. Me." I instructed.

Yes, I sucked at smoking pot in college. I'd take one hit and would get super paranoid and hide in a corner while my girlfriends were social butterflies, flirting with guys and dancing on tables. I'd then disappear to raid whatever food I could find, eat it all in a creepy silence, and then pass out. *So…who wants to party with me?*

Sitting outside of the restaurant, I could see fearful images appear in my mind: me fainting, lying on the floor, the sound of the sirens as the ambulance arrives, the rush to the ER, and the embarrassment of explaining my situation to doctors. I met each scary image with *not real, not real, not real…just breathe…feel the floor, the chair, the table…this is real.* Eventually the thoughts, feelings, and physical sensations passed.

The rest of the group joined us outside, and we laughed as we reminisced about the past and all of the hilarious things we did together in our twenties…and mostly how impressed we were that we all lived through it! Since one in eight women now get breast cancer, I let the gals know that I was taking one for the team.

Despite wigging out, I still had me some hair to wear home to hubby! Time for him to meet Samantha. I thought he'd like her. Our sex life had been…well…non-existent. It seemed my libido had peaced out along with my hair, so maybe this would help both of us. It did! But not for long.

Bodies don't think, care, or have any problem with themselves. They never beat themselves up or shame themselves. They simply try to keep themselves balanced and healthy. They're entirely efficient, intelligent, kind, and resourceful. When there's no thought, there's no problem.

—BYRON KATIE

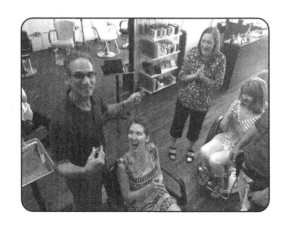

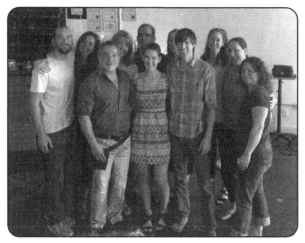

Hair Party

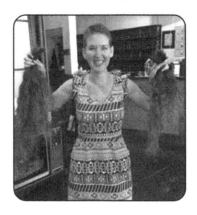

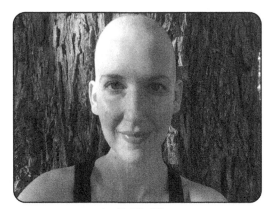

1st Baldie Photo

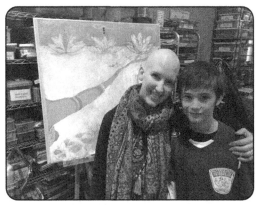

My Sweet, Nainoa

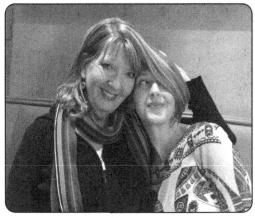

Wearing Mom's Hair

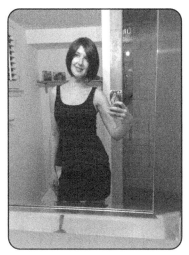

Samantha

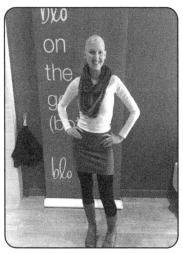

Bald is the New Beautiful

10

The Future of My Boobs
(FOMB)

"ARE YOU FUCKING CRAZY?" Travis's words were a dagger in my heart. "It's insane to even consider a double mastectomy."

"I'm not saying that's what I'm doing. I was just saying that I can see the benefits of getting one. I've been doing The Work on it, and I can really see good things in all surgery options. If I test positive for the breast cancer gene, the surgeon is going to recommend a double, so I'm just mentally preparing." *Jesus Christ, he is so intense. This is my body, not his. He really is turning into an ass about Western medicine!*

My Christmas gift came early: the test results were negative. *Thank God.* I really wanted a lumpectomy anyway, and now I could avoid more arguments with my husband. What happened to that whole "cancer makes our relationship stronger, I support you no matter what" vibe? I was not feeling it right now. *Ugh.* I brushed my frustrations aside as I prepared for my appointment with the breast surgeon. A little over halfway through chemo, this was the day we would learn the latest CT scan results, which would determine my surgery options.

A very clear movie played in my head about how I wanted this meeting to go down. It went like this: The surgeon swoops in with a huge smile on her face doing a happy dance and says, "Oh wow, we are all so blown away with your progress and the cancer is gone! And how great is it that you don't carry the gene for breast cancer either! No need to even consider a mastectomy. For surgery, we will only need to take a teensy weensy bit out to triple-check that the tissue is cancer-free. You won't even notice a difference in your beautiful breast. This will all be over before you know it and you can go back to making fun non-cancer-related plans in your life!"

As you can see, I was really good at practicing the art of non-attachment. Crap, now I was remembering how the last meeting with her went…how the treatment plan she laid out was way more complex than I expected and I had left the office with sea legs, terror, and tears. I started feeling uneasy about this next meeting. The "what if" worrying mind went back to work taking the past and projecting it into the future.

What if I am, again, naïve about what I think is a surgical option for me? What if I can't handle what she says to me? What if there's actually a chance I may lose my breast? It is so hard to love "what is" when you're stuck in a case of the "what-ifs."

After taking these thoughts to inquiry, a clear direction was presented. This was how I walked into the meeting: *my job is to show up, be open, ask questions, and the next step will be shown to me.*

Consulting with the breast surgeon this time was like meeting with a different person. She was full of smiles and relief. With the scan showing only microscopic signs of cancer, she was absolutely blown away by my progress. She told me I had literally "made her day" and was the success story she was telling to many of her other patients. *Look! I got what I imagined for this part! Perhaps I should consider a career in fortune telling after all.*

I did have all three surgery options, which was great news. However, the lumpectomy she described was not what I imagined. She could "try" to do a lumpectomy but would still need to take out all of the tissue that was originally affected by the cancer to make sure we got clear margins. When she held out a ruler, the amount of tissue to be removed looked to be the size of an orange. Furthermore, this procedure would leave my breast with a noticeable deformity, and it would not match the other breast. Radiation would shrink the breast further, making it more deformed and asymmetrical.

Unfortunately, my left breast was already smaller than my right one. *Dammit, universe, why didn't you cancer up my right boobie instead?* My heart sank.

Baffled, I asked, "According to the latest diagnostic tests, the cancer is already almost gone—so why take out so much tissue?" I learned that not all cancer cells show up in tests and since only the microscope can tell for sure, they remove all of the tissue that was originally affected. I continued to press, "What's the point of doing five months of intense chemo to shrink the tumor if you're basically going to take out the same amount of tissue anyways?"

She responded, "Think of the tumor as a glass mirror. When I throw it on the ground, it shatters into pieces. This is what the chemo is doing to the tumor— we hope that we are getting all of the shards, but they tend to spread out. You did have a few satellite nodules in other parts of your breast that were far away from the original tumor site. And I would be taking out less than we would have needed to in the beginning. Remember that cancer is a systemic disease, so the chemo's main goal is to kill the cancer cells in the entire body, and because we have seen how well your tumors have responded to the chemo, this tells us it is definitely working for the rest of the body too. This is good news! When you first came in and I saw the size of these tumors, I was really, really worried. So this is just amazing to see your response." Apparently, with a lumpectomy, there was a slightly greater statistical chance the cancer could come back and/or she might not be able to get clear margins, possibly requiring a second surgery.

From her perspective, a mastectomy was the safest option and the plastic surgeon—*holy shit...I might actually have a plastic surgeon?*—could make sure that the other breast looked even. The chances of cancer coming back would be decreased, and I wouldn't need an annual mammogram on my left breast.

Over time with aging, would my right boob grow down while the other stayed up? *Creepy.* And was it really true that there was nothing they could do to fill in the breast after a lumpectomy so that it wouldn't look deformed? Couldn't we just throw a sandbag in there (organic, vegan, and gluten-free of course)? How much radiation shrinkage were we talking about? Would I have a twelve-year-old's boob on one side?

A double mastectomy is usually what women my age do. That way, there is a decreased chance of recurrence, the breasts are both perky and even for life, and mammograms are no longer required for monitoring. According to my doctor, this procedure does not increase the survival rate but is more of an "emotional" deci-sion. I was not a candidate for using body fat to build the breasts since I didn't have enough of it, so implants would be used. #skinnybitchproblems

On top of all this, I was also going to need an axillary dissection surgery in my left armpit to remove the affected lymph nodes. Depending on the state of my pit, up to 35 nodes would be removed, putting me at risk for lymphedema.

Geez. This is a lot to take in. It's again, not what I expected. I guess I can kinda see bonuses and downsides for all three options, and hopefully at some point, something will stand out as a clear YES for me. It's just so crazy I'm even thinking about this!!! Dude, people my age are supposed to be focusing on having babies and/or growing their careers, not being forced to choose if they should remove body parts to avoid dying. It would probably be an easier decision if I didn't care what my boobs looked like or if I was super old…but yes, I'll admit it: I want the sexy bikini yogini bod back. Right now, I am a 108 pound bald stick figure. Is this vain? Maybe. And it's also honest.

Luckily, I was given plenty of time to make a decision, about two months, so I could finish chemo and give my body a little recovery time. After our meeting, I stood alone in the hospital hallway looking out the window at the heavy rain. The rain hardened into hail. While listening to the soft thumps of hail hitting the floor and metal railings, I was overcome with a comforting feeling of peace and pride.

My eyes started to tear up, and I just breathed it all in. *Damn, even though the meeting went differently than I anticipated, I handled it so well. And I wasn't trying to be strong, it happened naturally. Here I am, not knowing my decision, and I'm OK with it. OK with not knowing.* Cancer was continuing to teach me how to make peace with the unknown.

In the blink of an eye, two months flew by…*OK, decision, you can arrive now!* I still had no fucking clue what to do. I did, however, finish C-Love. *Woot! Woot!* After the last session, I rang that bell through tears of gratitude. Oh my God, it felt SO good to check a huge part of treatment off my list as "done." Right after the bell ringing, I made my shy family do the *Nae Nae* dance with me in front of the nurses and patients in the infusion room. And I got the video to prove it. Ah, the power of playing the C card.

Back to D-Day for surgery. I had really thought that all I would have to do was sit quietly in meditation and watch this clear beautiful neon sign of an answer flash before my eyes. Just in case I didn't see it, the sign would be accompanied by a deep, loving voice saying, "Bethany…you will have _____ surgery."

I joke, but this actually did happen once. When I moved back to the States after living in Spain, I was trying to determine my new career path. It was clear to me that advertising was no longer my calling, so what was next? I was taking one of my mom's yoga classes, and in the middle of a bridge pose, the craziest thing happened. I heard a voice—one that sounded just like mine—and it said as clear as day, "I'm going to be a yoga teacher." I heard my voice respond to it, "Yep, that's it." *What. Just. Happened.* But I was exhilarated; I couldn't wait for class to be over so I could tell my mom. I was literally shaking with excitement. "Mom, guess what?! I figured out what I'm going to do next—I'm going to be a yoga teacher!" Her response was so amusing, "That's a great job to have while you're figuring out what you really want to do in life!" Ahhhhh…nearly ten years later, it was still a career I absolutely loved.

Unfortunately, no number of bridge poses has resurrected that damn beautiful, clear God-like voice. My "peace with the unknown" expired quickly. In fact, the whole "decision-making" process was the most challenging, gut-wrenching, emotional part of this entire journey thus far. There were times I wished I didn't have a choice. I had even wished the cancer would show up somewhere else in my left breast or even in my other breast so I could know what to do.

Why did this suck? What made this so excruciatingly diffi- cult? I was believing the thought (insert dramatic music here)... *I will make the wrong decision.*

Under the influence of this thought, I became paralyzed with fear. My mind could only see the worst-case scenarios for each option. *It's all shit and I'm forced to choose from the lesser of three evil shits.* In this space, I really did feel like a victim, furious that I was in this situation. I wanted someone or something to give me a clear answer. I worried what people would think of me and told myself that I was a failure at being "peaceful." Overcome with emotions, I tightened my body, leading to exhaustion, achier muscles, and headaches. Headaches so often, in fact, that the oncologist ordered a brain MRI to make sure the cancer hadn't spread to my brain. In summary, when I believed this thought, I felt like complete, total, and utter crap.

Without the thought, I was so much lighter. The pressure was lifted (literally) off my shoulders, and I could see and focus on the blessings in each option. I felt more motivated to take action. Possibilities filled my mind: I could gather more information, get second opinions, talk to other survivors, sit with myself, and enjoy living my life. I now felt empowered, open, free, and trusting of my own intuition and the universe. *What if it's not possible for me to do it wrong?*

Had I ever really made a "wrong" decision? Even the times I had thought something bad was happening, it had turned out to be even better than I imagined. I broke my ankle and met my husband… we were almost kicked out of our home and ended up moving to a retreat property and creating a new business…I failed my first yoga training and then started my own private practice. I got cancer and it ended up being a gift in many ways. The only thing that could go "wrong" was the big W sticky note my mind put on it. *I will make the right decision* was truer. Whatever decision I made *was* the right decision, the right path for me. *Hmmmm….I'm feeling much better.*

Here are some other stressful thoughts I took to inquiry during my decision-making process: *People will judge me. If I choose a lumpectomy, the cancer will come back. If I choose a double, I will not like my breasts. I should be more peaceful in this process. I want the universe to give me a clear decision. I am not "evolved" if I choose a double mastectomy.*

Doing The Work truly helped to bring me back to the present moment and clear my mind of some majorly bogus myths. Still, I would fluctuate between attaching and unattaching from some of those thoughts. Here are a few more techniques that supported me in finding a clear answer…maybe my possibly psycho over-the-top processing approach will serve you in some way when you're faced with a tough decision.

Clarifying My Intention

Sitting with the questions *Why am I choosing surgery? What is its purpose? What do I want from this experience in the long term?* helped me to determine a clear vision to hold as I walked through different options. For me, it boiled down to: (1) Cure this body of cancer cells. (2) Prevent cancer cells from returning. (3) Feel long-term mental peace. (4) Look and feel good about my body.

Gathering Information

I dove into learning as much as possible about each option, consulting Web MD and Google images. Just kidding! DON'T DO THIS! Ahhhhh! Instead, I asked more questions of my breast and plastic surgeon, got second opinions, and spoke with other women who had chosen each type of surgery.

I learned a ton. A much less invasive lumpectomy was an option according to my second-opinion breast surgeon. Instead of taking out a chunk of tissue the size of an orange from my breast, she would aim to take out a cherry's worth. (Did I just ruin fruit for you?) What I had originally wanted was actually possible! Yippee! Of course, clear margins were necessary, which could lead to more surgeries. There was also a higher risk of recurrence with a lumpectomy; a double mastectomy would reduce the recurrence rate in the breast from 12% to 1%.

For a lumpectomy, "You get what you get" in terms of how the breast would look was not true. There were plastic surgery techniques to help the breasts look even. In a separate surgery, the other breast could be reduced and lifted to match the cancer side, which involved cutting out the nipple and moving it up. *Ewwww… creepy.* Lumpectomies also required more monitoring of the breast tissue using frequent mammograms and ultrasounds.

For a single mastectomy, the plastic surgeon could also make the other side match. However, over time, aging would make the real breast sag while the other remained the same. There was always the option of getting more plastic surgery, I supposed.

A single or double mastectomy would involve at least two surgeries. The first one removes the breast tissue, and expanders are put in place underneath the pectoral muscles to help stretch the skin and prepare the breasts for radiation and the final implants. The implants would be inserted eight to twelve months after radiation, and extra fat would be injected between the implants and the skin for a more natural look and feel. *Holy torpedo Batman, that seems like forrrrrever.*

My first-opinion plastic surgeon recommended a combination of taking fat from my belly and implants, leaving a massive hip-to-hip scar and a third surgery. Thank God, my second opinion plastic surgeon put one hand on my stomach and said, "I wouldn't touch this." He offered a less invasive technique for reconstruction that included the use of implants plus liposuction from my love handles. Less scarring, less surgery, and an easier recovery. After double mastectomies, there would be no more mammograms or ultrasounds, only the occasional chest X-ray or breast MRI.

Given that cancer was found in my lymph nodes, radiation was recommended regardless of the surgery I chose.

OK, brain. Two things were now clear: (1) I preferred my second-opinion medical team, and (2) because of gravity, doing a single mastectomy was not an option for me. It would have to be either a lumpectomy or a double. *I can't believe I am actually considering a double mastectomy.*

Throughout this entire journey, I had been sharing my experience, fears, and inner work on my blog and Facebook. I realized it might be crazy to hash out my decision-making process in front of an audience. Maybe it would have been more intelligent to withhold sharing until I'd made a decision so that I didn't unintentionally invite in hundreds of other people's opinions. With so many other opinions floating around (and there had been many throughout this whole process!), it was sometimes hard to hear my own voice. Yet, I wanted to remain an open book, so I shared anyway with this clear message: I love you and I'm not sharing this information to get your opinion on what I should do for my body.

Online, I explained that it can be very easy to have a clear opinion on treatment when you have *never* been in this situation. I knew, because this used to be me. Before I experienced any of this, I would have said, "People are crazy to even consider chemo and to remove a breast or two is even crazier!"

Dude, my Guru Cancer, had totally humbled me and kicked me off of my judgmental, arrogant high horse. Thank goodness this experience had opened my mind to seeing the truth: there is no single "right" way of dealing with cancer treatment. There are many "right" ways. What's right for you may not be right for me, and that's so OK. I don't know what's best for anyone else, ever. Treatment is a super-personal decision, and I'll no longer judge how anyone else chooses to heal.

Who do I really want to hear from right now? Women who had been there. There is an instant bond that exists with cancer thrivers—an immediate sense of connection and compassion. Each woman I connected with gave me the same helpful reminder that it was completely normal to feel everything I was feeling. Fear, worry, anxiety, doubt…these are all natural human emotions in life and in this process. I am not alone. Ever. This was so comforting.

I had the opportunity to ask them lots of questions. "Are you happy with your surgical decision? How has your life been affected? Would you do anything differently? Did you keep your nipples? How is sex now?"

For some of the women who chose a lumpectomy, the cancer returned, and they ended up getting a mastectomy or a double. The ones who were very happy with their lumpectomy and were still cancer-free had a much smaller tumor initially with no involvement of the lymph nodes. For the double-mastectomy women, most of them told me that the procedure was hard but not as tough as they thought it would be, and not one person regretted their decision.

Everyone reminded me that I needed to do what felt right for me.

Many weeks into this information-gathering phase, I again started to get completely overwhelmed…I was hoping that during one of the meetings, something would just click and my decision would be made. But I still felt torn.

One late afternoon, I was lying in bed when my husband walked in. "Hey honey, do you want a salad with dinner? If so, I'll run up to Whole Foods and buy lettuce." Instead of seeing how thoughtful this question was and realizing that *holy crap—my husband is actually cooking me dinner tonight*, I completely lost it. "I don't know! YOU make the decision! I can't handle it!" I pulled the covers over my head and sobbed.

Yeah…it was definitely time to take a break and step away from everything. I attempted to focus on just living and enjoying my life and my boobs. Then Type A Bethany took over with…

The Good Ol' Pro/Con List

I'm a dork at heart. I created an entire spreadsheet titled "The Future of My Boobs (FOMB)" listing the pros and cons of each surgery option, along with the procedure recommended by each doctor and additional questions and things to consider. I scheduled a FOMB meeting with Mom and Travis to walk through everything together. At this point, chemo brain was in full effect, so this process helped me to better organize my thoughts and make sure I had a clear understanding of each option.

Speaking of chemo brain…there's a debate about whether or not chemo brain is real. Let me tell you, this shit be real! My mind had become total mush on so many occasions, forgetting dates, names, conversations, where I was, or why I opened the fridge. Sometimes I stood in the grocery aisle and asked myself, "Why am I here?" until a box of crackers spoke to me.

But chemo brain never stressed me out. Do you know why? Because I didn't believe the thought *I should be able to remember.* I just trusted the information would come to me if it was meant to. I wasn't too shy to ask others for help if I forgot something either. I had also become really good at putting reminders and alerts into my phone.

Cancer patients are dealing with a buttload of new information all of the time on top of living an actual life with responsibilities AND dealing with big emotions and physical challenges. So we deserve to forget—there ain't no shame in it. Plus, how often have you wished that you could be completely and totally present? Not remembering has its gifts.

OK, back to my never-ending decision-making process. Next up, I went for a more feely approach.

Trying It On & Feeling It Out

I decided to "try on" my two different decisions as if I were trying on a new dress. *OK, I'm doing a lumpectomy. How does it feel? Do I notice any physical sensations? How do I feel as I imagine the next 60 years?* Then I tried on the double.

I was stunned. When I tried on a lumpectomy…I lost my breath and constricted my body, feeling extremely anxious. When I tried on a double, I felt relief.

What?! This is not what I expected to feel. I mean, after all, I had ended up getting what I thought I wanted with a less invasive lumpectomy, the cherry! But the truth was, it still didn't feel right. A lumpectomy seemed easier this year, but harder in the long run with the constant monitoring of my lumpy-ass breast tissue. Remember how many lumps I had before cancer? I had no idea if I would ever have cancer again, but I was pretty confident that I would have lumps again, and I would want to get each one thoroughly investigated.

A double mastectomy appeared harder at that moment, since it extended my treatment plan by a whole year, but I felt so much more at ease as I imagined the rest of my life.

I also noticed that when I talked to people about it, I was looking for them to tell me it was OK to choose a double mastectomy. Geez, there was even that moment of hoping for more cancer to show up so I could make this decision. Instead of looking outward for this permission, I decided to give it to myself instead.

So yes, I chose to do a double mastectomy. *O.M.G.*

I was utterly terrified to tell Hubby. This was his favorite part of my body and an important aspect of our sex life. And I was unnecessarily removing it. Well, it was necessary for my peace of mind, but he might not see it that way. It was also going against what we had discussed in the beginning of this process. In addition, he had already admitted that he was not attracted to "fake boobs." Then again, he had finally started to practice The Work more often on his own. Hopefully it had rubbed off a bit on him.

To soften the blow, I took him to our favorite spot by Turtle Creek, the spot where we spontaneously moon married ourselves six years ago. We sat on a wool yoga blanket cross-legged facing each other. I felt a gentle breeze blowing under the rose-colored scarf covering my bald head. I held his hands as I told him, "I've made a decision about the surgery. I'm going to have a double mastectomy." He paused a moment, then laughed. "Were you afraid to tell me or something?"

"Ummmm…YES! Can you blame me?" He looked lovingly into my eyes and uttered the exact words I wanted to hear, "OK. I understand. If this is what you really want, I'll support you." My heart melted into him. *What a relief.* As the sun set, we nestled under the blanket by the creek and watched the fireflies dance over the water.

In the days leading up to my surgery, my mind did not always stay clear and calm. I began to enter a mental ping-pong match of second guessing EVERYTHING. *Am I making a mistake? Will I regret it? Are these just pre-surgery jitters or is this my heart talking?*

All I wanted was that feeling of clarity to come back and stay forever. *Is it true?* Or did I want the opportunity to be with myself in these deep emotions? After all, I was going through what seemed like a natural and necessary grieving process for my breasts.

Within seconds I could go from feeling perfectly fine to sobbing. Sleep didn't come easily, and I would wake up in the middle of the night in tears. Movement helped—longer walks, jumping on the trampoline, yoga, Epsom salt baths.

One day, in a fit of anger, I tore up a cardboard box. I also attended an incredible Somatic Movement and Sound Healing Workshop, crying before, a little during, and a ton afterwards. I spent some time sketching pictures of my breasts, which was healing, along with talking to them, caressing them, and thanking them for being such a big part of my life.

My breasts will never be the same as they once were. Well, actually, they were already not the same. They resembled long test tubes now that chemo had deflated the hell out of them. They had even earned a medical term: *breast ptosis*. I couldn't imagine that aging would help that situation. So how did I know they wouldn't be *better*? The worst that could happen was my stressful story about them. It was comforting to know I always had inquiry.

But I am losing my breasts! Wait—was I really? Or was it truer that in reality, I was simply having breast tissue, tissue that I had *never* even actually seen or touched because it was under my skin, replaced with a material that was less likely to grow cancer? *I am gaining my breasts.* Yes, new cancer-free, anti-gravity boobs. And just like that, I popped back into the clarity and peace that I was making the right decision.

We never make a decision. When the time is right, the decision makes itself.

—BYRON KATIE

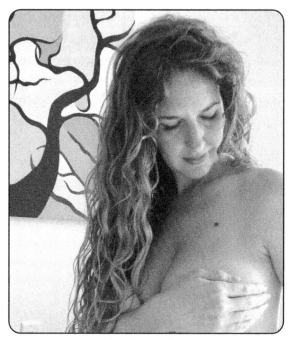

Bye Bye Boobies

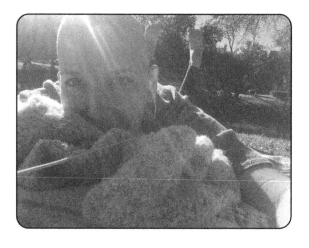

11

Gratitude, Elephants, & Going Potty: Breast Surgery

FACEBOOK UPDATE

Walking into tomorrow's surgery, I am simply filled with gratitude. I am grateful for the expertise, compassion, and care of the surgical team, nurses, pathologists, assistants, administrators, and volunteers who will take me into their arms tomorrow.

I am thankful I feel an unwavering trust in their abilities while my body comfortably rests on the operating table. I am thankful for the needles, medicine, bed, warm blankets, machines, drains, and tubing that will allow me to feel relaxed and supported. I am grateful for the knives and other surgical tools that will further clear this body of cancer cells.

I am grateful for all of the women who have walked this path before me—allowing for improvements in research, technology, and healthcare so that I can experience the highest outcome of healing. I am grateful for my family staying with me in this journey through all of the ups and downs.

I am thankful for YOU and the consistent kind words of support and encouragement. I truly feel you with me, and I love that we can connect like this. I am thankful for my beautiful breasts and the 34 years of fun we have experienced together; I am grateful to soon receive new breasts and look forward to our adventures.

I am grateful to myself for really diving in and showing up for each and every gift of this process. And I am thankful to cancer for teaching me kindness, compassion, resilience, strength, trust, and acceptance. It has cracked me wide open (pun intended).

I welcome fear, and at this moment, I simply cannot find it. Just love. Thank you for being

with me tomorrow. My sweet mamma will be
posting updates.

I love you,
Bethany

The Facebook comments kept pouring in, each one tugging
at my heartstrings. Such a collective feeling of oneness. People
are so kind.

That night, my husband, Mom, and I sat in a circle, lit a candle,
and listened to a pre-surgery meditation. Eyes closed, I snuck
a quick peek at two of my favorite people. *I am so lucky.* Before
closing my eyes again, I caught a glimpse of the moonlight glistening over the oak trees outside my sliding glass window. When
it ended, we sat in silence, eyes glistening with tears. It may sound
cheesy, but it was a really special moment. I was just amazed. I
mean wow, I had not expected that I would ever get to that level of
clarity. A complete calm had washed over me. *I. Am. Just. So. Ready.*
This is awesome! Can I bottle up this feeling so it can last forever?

The next morning, my alarm rang at 4:45am. I woke to pitch
blackness, hearing the rain pouring outside. Oddly, I felt excitement. This early awakening reminded me of going on road trips as
a kid. My parents would wake us up at the butt crack of dawn. Still
half asleep and in pajamas, we'd pile into the car. I'd have a rush of
Woohoo, a new adventure! excitement before falling right back asleep.
Yes, my parents were smart, as this gave them a few hours of peaceful
silence before the three of us started chanting "Are we there yet? I'm
bored! He's bothering me!" Hey, this was life before iPads.

And now here we were, another new adventure. I hopped in
the shower and washed myself with the smelly pink antibiotic soap
provided by the surgeon, taking time to feel the full sensations of

my breasts for the last time. *Gosh I'm going to miss this. And that's OK.* I dressed in comfy, loose clothing I could easily put back on after my surgery with my soon-to-be T-Rex arms. We gathered in the dimly lit kitchen, hospital bags in hand…*let's do this!*

I felt this same blend of peace/excitement/curiosity in each moment leading up to surgery, even declining the nurse's offer to take a Xanax and some poop drugs before the procedure. *Oh yeah, I am so evolved. I don't need those stinkin' drugs.*

There was one moment when I lost my cool. Upon our arrival in the pre-op room, the nurse walked in and asked, "OK, Bethany, what are you having done today?" My first reaction was *Well, uhhh….shouldn't YOU know that?! Why are YOU asking ME? Panic, holy shit, they are so flipping disorganized, you have to be kidding me, how am I supposed to trust them with my body and this HUGE surgery if they don't even know what the F I'm here for!?!?*

Then I learned that this is standard protocol…hehehehe…. They are required to ask you this question when you arrive, and I would be asked the same question over and over again by each nurse, volunteer, the breast surgeon, plastic surgeon, anesthesiologist, small children, strangers passing by…until I drifted off into my peaceful slumber. I laughed at my mind as I realized that they were all doing this to be helpful, efficient, and avoid mistakes. And hey, oh goodie—I knew the answer to the question!

"I am here for a nipple-sparing bilateral mastectomy. The breast surgeon will also remove the chemo port, and in the left axilla, she will perform a sentinel node biopsy, with a possible lymph node dissection. The plastic surgeon will insert tissue expanders, with a possible allograft." Look! I could speak medical now!

Here is my procedure translated into plain English:

- **Nipple Sparing:** I would get to keep my nipples. Because the original cancer was a good distance away from my nipple, I was a candidate for nipple conservation. However, this was not guaranteed. The surgeon would swipe a sample of the tissue from underneath each nipple and test it to confirm there were no microscopic cancer cells. If cancer was found, it would be bye-bye nipples. There was also a chance the blood flow to the nipples would not work properly or that the skin could die.

- **Bilateral Mastectomy:** The removal of all breast tissue (and cancer!) in both of my breasts.

- **Chemo Port:** This was the medical device that was inserted during a day surgery before I began chemotherapy—my superhero plug. *It's been great, but I don't need you anymore, peace out!*

- **Sentinel Node Biopsy:** This was a standard procedure involving identifying, removing, and examining the sentinel nodes (the first few lymph nodes closest to the breast) for any signs of cancer. A dye would be injected into the axilla (armpit area) that turns a certain color if something is cancerous. Usually between one and three lymph nodes are removed.

- **Lymph Node Dissection:** If the above procedure showed cancer, this procedure would be done, which involves removing additional lymph nodes and some of the surrounding tissue. The average is twelve lymph nodes, but this process could even result in all of them being removed depending on what the surgeon saw. (NOTE: My surgeon leaned more towards the conservative side, as there was a good deal of recent research confirming that taking out fewer lymph nodes led to fewer complications, and radiation could clean up any remaining cancer cells).

- **Tissue Expanders:** After the breast surgeon performed the above procedures, the plastic surgeon would replace the breast tissue with tissue expanders underneath the pectoral muscles. These hard balloon-like temporary implants would slowly be filled with saline over the next six to eight weeks after the surgery to help stretch the skin and prepare the boobies for radiation and the final breast reconstruction surgery.

- **Allograft:** If the tissue expanders did not fit securely underneath the pectoral muscles, the plastic surgeon would add extra tissue (allograft) to help them stay in place. The tissue comes from donors—no, not creepy at all—and is deeply cleaned and processed so no DNA remains. Think of it as extra boobie padding. From dead people.

Going into surgery, I was in complete surrender to the unknown. I remembered that during my pre-op visits with my surgeons, I had asked them the best way to prepare for surgery. "The best thing to prepare is your mind. Trust us. We have your best interests in mind and we want the best possible outcome for you." I was so blown away by the awesomeness of these doctors and of conventional medicine. I continued to see proof that my beliefs about conventional medicine were wrong. Doctors are connected, kind, intelligent, and experienced.

Byron Katie often talks about how there are only three Types of Business in the world—mine, yours, and God's. So whose business was my cancer? Not mine. I loved that I could hand my body, my cancer, over to doctors. To people who had much more experience with cancer cells than I did. Healing cancer was their job, not mine. I also surrendered to the Universe because there was something greater at work here that was beyond all of our control. That was God's business. *God, another word for reality, will show us the way. I'm not in charge of healing myself. What a relief!* This freed me up to focus on my job, my business: heal my mind and enjoy the ride.

In the pre-op room, I became child-like and curious. It was so cool! *Did they secretly give me Xanax or something? How in the hell am I this calm?* Each person who walked in was smiling and kind. I marveled in wonder while the plastic surgeon drew artistic lines all over my chest with a red marker. His eyes met mine with a reassuring confidence, "You're OK. We've got this." And yes, he was wearing cowboy boots with his scrubs. This was Texas after all!

My breast surgeon looked focused and well rested as she twisted her long, wavy hair up into a bun. *This is what they do and they do it well.* I watched the fluids enter into my arm. I saw the care and concern in my husband's and mother's eyes. Neither wanted to leave my side. My last hug and kiss with each of them was special and intimate, not scary.

I found this out later and thought it was just so cool. Before the procedure began, my breast surgeon went to find my mother. She pointed out a special place to sit in the waiting room. "Your daughter will be on the operating table just on the other side of this same wall. This is where you can be the closest to her." Wow. Pure kindness.

Time to move to the operating room. *I love being wheeled around in a bed! I'm now in a bed in an elevator! OK, this is definitely the drugs talking.* We busted through the operating room doors, and I was placed underneath these huge, bubbly lights that looked like colorful honeycombs. "Wow…these lights are so beautiful!" And that was it. Goodnight.

After eight hours of memory-less sleep, I woke up in a recovery room crowded with other patients, all separated by pale blue hospital curtains. *Holy ouch.* An intense, painful pressure on my chest hit me. *Is a giant elephant sitting on me?* Unable to fully breathe, I took small, shallow breaths while trying to focus on breathing into my belly. *Sahara desert. In my mouth.* The nurse seemed harried and overworked, but whenever I managed to get her attention with a wiggle of my index finger, I requested ice chips. *More, please.* The cold, wet, arctic liquid soothed every inch of my mouth and throat. As I floated in and out of consciousness, I could hear the moaning and groaning of other patients, and of one woman in particular. "Nurse! Nurse! It hurts! It hurts soooo much. Help me, please." *Wait—or is that me?*

I was wheeled into my final recovery room where we would stay for the next two nights, a private one with a view full of evergreen tress and an old crusty pull-out couch for Mom. I watched my husband, mom, and mother-in-law rush in to see me. Travis reached for my hand, "Hey baby, how are you?!" I smiled and replied, "OK. It's hard to breathe. It hurts. A lot." *Dang, it hurts way more than I thought it would, to be honest.* I still felt like I couldn't get a full breath. To help expand my lungs, a nurse handed me a device that looked like a giant penis pump from Austin Powers, instructing me to blow hard into it. *Lol…really?*

"Here is your morphine pain pump. If you feel pain, pump it every eight minutes when the green light turns on," the nurse explained. Some of the other women I had talked to who had gone through this surgery had told me that they hadn't even needed the pain pump or maybe only used it once. Well…I pumped that shit like it was a hand Jazzercise class. Later that evening when it still hadn't seemed to relieve the freaking pain, they asked me if I wanted a morphine boost. All of the *I'm so evolved and awesome and don't need extra medicine* bullshit thoughts vanished, replaced with: *YES, PLEASE. GIVE ME DRUGS.*

On top of the pain, we soon encountered an unexpected and uncommon side effect of the anesthesia: I couldn't pee. I sat on the toilet again and again…I pressed on my stomach, let water run in the faucet, put my hand in hot water, listened to waterfall music from Mom's iPhone, counted tiles to distract my mind… nothing worked! The internal pressure continued to build until I was pregnant with a pee baby. *Looks like I get to have a baby after all—too soon for infertility jokes?* What's cool about modern medicine is if you can't pee on your own, they can do it for you! I was catheterized…three times. Each time, they removed about a liter and a half of urine. The mild discomfort of a tube going up my you-know-what was nothing compared to the sweet Jesus relief I experienced when it was over.

After the second day in the hospital, I finally began to pee on my own, a victory greater than reaching the peak of Mount Everest. Talk about learning to appreciate the simple things in life we take for granted. *I can peeeeeeeeeeee!*

Which leads me to my next teaching moment…If you are ever in the presence of someone who cannot pee, here are three things *not* to say or do: (1) "Just try harder." (2) "We really need you to be able to go to the bathroom on your own." (3) If I politely ask for everyone to leave the room so I can try to pee in solitude, LEAVE THE ROOM instead of standing close enough to me so that my knee is brushing the back of your thigh while I'm on the toilet. Especially if we just met 30 seconds ago.

All jokes aside, the staff was amazing. Even though the pain level was so much more intense than I had expected, there were many moments when that pain was completely non-existent: when I heard a joke, watched a show on Netflix, when the nurses asked me what I wanted for lunch, when my husband kissed me on the forehead, when I was fast asleep. When my attention was elsewhere, there was no pain. *Whoa.* So where did the pain go in those moments? *This is freaking fascinating, isn't it?*

My mind was also open to recognizing the reality that so many things were actually BETTER than I had anticipated. For example, the moment when I saw my new breasts. Before surgery, I had dreaded that moment. I had imagined it on so many occasions and was brought to tears every time. I pictured myself standing before the hospital mirror, seeing the first glimpse of my creepy-looking-mutilated-used-to-be-beautiful-and-never-will-be-again breasts. Then horror and regret would fill my mind.

On Day 2, I lifted up my gown, looked in the mirror, and was pleasantly surprised. "Wow—they look pretty damn good for just coming out of surgery! Hey honey, did you see these?" I now had adorable little A-cup breasts. The incisions were along the outer and lower part of each breast, and I still had nipples! The clear surgical tape was wrapped around me like a bra. Oddly, my now-purple nips were squeezing out of the tape to increase blood flow. *OK, that's kinda weird.* I could see some swelling and discoloring from bruising, which was expected. There was also some discoloring in my husband's face…poor guy, his favorite part of my body had just been replaced. #husbandsdeservetogrievetoo

OK, so it was creepy as hell that there were tubes poking out of my body, draining blood and excess fluid into these little hand pumps I got to clean out every day.

But OMG, I could still feel some areas of my breasts! I had heard that you can lose all of your sensation, which had made me anxious. Sensation meant a lot to me personally and sexually with my husband. I did hear from another woman that yes, she did lose sensation but "other senses are heightened if you know what I mean…wink, wink." I could still feel about 40% of my boobies—yeah!

After two days of recovery and proving I could walk and pee on my own, I was wheeled out of the hospital with my stuffed donkey and flowers in hand and entrusted to my two primary caregivers: Hubby Travis and Superwoman Mommy.

When you're asleep, does your body hurt? When you're in the worst pain and the phone rings and it's the call you've been waiting for and you're mentally focused on the phone call, there's no pain. If you change your thinking, you change the pain.

—BYRON KATIE

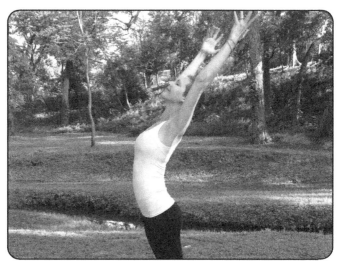

Day Before Surgery

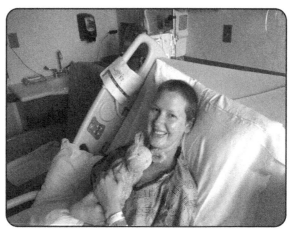

Post Surgery

12

Self-Discovery While in Recovery

THE FIRST TEN DAYS OF RECOVERY were packed with ups and downs. There were moments of "Fuck this shit, I'd rather die than feel this pain anymore" and moments of "Wow, I have never felt this loved and supported." The whole experience turned out to be quite the invitation to explore stressful thoughts that had held me back from self-love.

Every single nerve-racking story about medicine and pain returned with a vengeance. *Oh really, you think you got this pain thing down? You think you're totally OK with medicine? I'll show you biatch!!!* The physical pain was so freaking intense that I could not see anything other than *ouch…it hurts. Help. Ouch. It hurts. So bad. It will seriously never go away. Make it stop. Please.*

And then I noticed something underneath, something even

more painful: *I feel like a complete and utter failure. I shouldn't be in so much pain. I should be handling this more peacefully.* If I took medicine, I'd hate myself. If I didn't take medicine, I'd love myself but be in pain. My self-love was completely conditional. These self-admonishing thoughts kept multiplying until...

I had no choice but to surrender. Surrender "working on myself," "being evolved," "being peaceful at healing." *Screw it. Take the drugs, lady!* What? Those drugs aren't working? Increase the dosage. Go back to the doctor. Take different drugs. Sleep. Cry. What? It hurts like hell to cry or cough? You feel like you're being stabbed in the heart when you sneeze? Good. Do it anyways because that's what's happening. What? Your mind is distracted and doesn't feel as much pain while binge-watching Netflix? Awesome. Watch more.

Why can't all of this be self-love too? I wouldn't judge others for having a hard time in recovery—why am I so tough on myself?

So once I got over myself, which was actually me getting over my story of how I should be doing this recovery thing, I was able to love myself without conditions and open my mind to the blessings of this part of the journey.

For example, even being in pain, there were so many things I was capable of doing! I could go on (slow-motion) walks, eat amazing meals, spend time with my family, crack jokes, sing karaoke, have deep heartfelt conversations, and post messages and pics on Facebook. Yes, it would take about 90 minutes to get ready for the day, but I was still doing it: shower, put on clothes, apply make-up, clean my drains. Daily acts turned into mindful meditation. Plus, I wasn't in pain 100% of the time. There were still those moments when I didn't even notice it.

On Day 10, I decided to take over-the-counter Midol® for my pain because the hardcore stuff didn't seem to be working as well as

I thought it would. Midol had worked best for my migraines in the past, and it ended up being my MIRACLE DRUG. It alleviated my chest pain within thirty minutes, and for the first time in ten days, relief and hope rushed in. There was a light at the end of the post-mastectomy tunnel.

Throughout the entire process, there was a warm and tender noticing. I was completely reconnecting with my inner child. I loved asking someone (most frequently Mom and Travis) to hold my hand. I asked to be cuddled. To be petted. Right then, that intimacy was my favorite thing in the entire world. It was so comforting and soothing to fall into someone's arms. And guess what? They were always happy to do it. When I was alone, I hugged my stuffed donkey and blanket. Yes, I was 34 years old and freaking loving being a baby again.

I also got to witness my superhuman-caretaker-of-the-year mom in full force! I started every morning lying in bed, yelling "Moooooooooommmm!" She would soon arrive with crackers, water, and meds, anticipating every need before I even knew I had one. She cooked for me, cleaned the house, held me, helped me vent and cry, and was truly there for me in my darkest moment.

At one point we realized that I was completely full of shit. Literally. Six days' worth of meals had yet to exit my body…constipation being one of the medicines' side effects. *Crap (pun intended), why didn't I accept those poop drugs in the hospital?* Let's just say after an evening of agony, tears, doing yoga over a toilet, bargaining with God to please just let me poop, Mom came to the rescue with a morning enema. I mean, seriously—is that unconditional love or what?

Luckily, Travis was out of town at a Byron Katie event in California for this sexy experience. I was ecstatic that he was finally saying yes to self-care. Plus, Nurse Mom was way more equipped to handle this part.

A few days later, after picking up a vegan pizza from Whole Foods, Mom was driving me to Klyde Warren Park in downtown Dallas for lunch. The breast surgeon called. We quickly pulled over. In a surprisingly sterile voice, she told us, "We got the pathology report back and there was 10mm of cancer left in your breast and 1.2cm left in your lymph nodes. We got clear margins so there is no evidence of disease." *Wait—is she saying what I think she is saying? The cancer is gone?* I asked her to clarify, and she said yes. We hung up the phone, bursting into sobs. I immediately called Travis, and we all sobbed some more.

This was the moment I had been waiting for since I got the "you have cancer" phone call eight months ago. But something was off. I wasn't as ecstatic as I had thought I would be. *I don't get it.* Instead of celebrating, my mind immediately jumped into the future, seeing how much more treatment there was to come… recovery, the tissue-expanding process, six weeks of radiation, reconstruction, hormone therapy…*Ugh.* It felt like so much. This was far from over. And instead of celebrating the fact that there was only 10mm of cancer left in my boobie, I turned on myself. *I had both breasts replaced for only 10mm of cancer?* Then my mind focused on the way the surgeon delivered the news, wondering why she wasn't more excited. *And why do doctors say "no evidence of disease" or "remission"? Why can't they just tell me I'm "cured"?*

Wow, minds can really suck the joy out of anything! I caught mine trying to ruin this moment. And I wasn't going to let it. Not this time! *The cancer is gone! I'm cured! Wahoooooooo!* Mom and I sat in the park to eat our now-celebratory pizza, watching the crowds of playing children, laughing families, and food trucks. Here I was, rocking a patchy Sinead O'Connor buzz cut and new expander boobs held by a bra full of tape under my loose shirt, with two drains comfortably concealed in my fanny pack. Not to mention that we had just found out that I didn't have cancer anymore. I smiled and looked at Mom. Not one person here knew what we had just been through. It was our sweet little secret.

Travis returned all blissed out from Byron Katie, and it was time for Mom to leave. My anxiety started up again. I worried about how my recovery would be with Travis at home with *I'm a burden to him* as my strongest belief. Plus, I was taking four weeks off of work, putting even more financial pressure on him after our relationship had already been tested so many other times in this journey.

Despite my fears, the turnaround, *I'm not a burden to him*, turned out to be more true. He expressed feeling that it was his honor to help me in this way and be there for me. For him, doing things for me and paying for things was his way of loving me. He hadn't always been able to be there for me during cancer treatment in the way we both would have wanted, so this was also an opportunity for him to make amends and for me to accept his loving support.

Working full-time, helping with Nainoa, and taking care of me was a lot of work, so I also began to outsource some tasks, especially when someone offered. In fact, I was getting pretty damn good at this "say yes" to help thing! I learned to get really specific when someone offered help: Are you able to bring me lunch tomorrow? Can you please drop off your adorable dog for dog therapy? Will you go for a walk with me? Are you available to give me a ride? Can you do The Work with me?

People are so kind. They want to help. It feels good to help. I know this because that's how I feel when I do things for others. It's why I love my job so much. Well, recovery was definitely a time for me to say yes to being on the receiving end. After all, "Let yourself be pampered by others" was literally written in the doctor's orders.

It was hilarious to see how creative and resourceful I could be. I discovered that I could open the fridge and dishwasher with my feet. My core strength helped me sit up and lie down. If Travis left the frying pan on the stove, I could cook simple meals. I asked him to put my morning juices and nut milks in smaller bottles that I could lift. It also helped that I lived within walking distance of fantastic restaurants and Whole Foods. I ditched the penis pump breathing device, replacing it with a new ritual of singing karaoke multiple times a day to expand my lungs … apparently I have an affinity for Disney songs, especially *Frozen*'s "Let It Go" and *Aladdin*'s "A Whole New World." Even Disney was dishing out great advice for recovery.

About two-and-a-half weeks after surgery, I received a very special gift from Shelby, a client and dear friend. It was a small plant with a green gem-like stone hanging over it. Shelby shared that she had searched all over for it and thought it was perfect for what I was going through. I assumed the green stone had some kind of cool healing property and set it on my granite kitchen island.

I was only now really starting to feel better physically, mentally, and emotionally. The pain became very manageable, and I was starting to move and groove with my arms again.

The next morning, I walked into the kitchen and froze. Delicately chilling in the plant was a huge gorgeous monarch butterfly. My entire being lit up in excitement. *Oh my God, what is this? Where did it come from?* That green "stone"? It was a butterfly cocoon!

Shelby didn't know this, but I have a deep love for butterflies. I have always felt a special connection with them. In eighth grade, I wrote a poem titled, "Life as a Butterfly," accompanied by a drawing of a woman with butterfly wings.

I think of myself as a butterfly,
First hiding inside of my tiny cocoon,
Then breaking through under the misty moon.
But first…
I was a vulnerable caterpillar,
Crawling along…
Humming the melody of my song,
Slowly changing and maturing,
I soon realize…
That I am no longer wearing a disguise,
For I have become visible to the world's eye.
I have become a beautiful butterfly.
I flutter from place to place,
Forgetting that the world is a disgrace
Until I finally land in a place full of wonders,
A land where I can call my own,
My own home.
I think of myself as a butterfly,
Waiting to spread my wings,
Listen to the glorious songs I shall sing.
For I will try…
So sit back and watch me fly!

Isn't she sweet? Not sure why the world was a disgrace at age fourteen, though. Maybe I had run out of allowance money and couldn't buy a new shirt at Contempo? Oh yeah—back to butter-flies. For our wedding, we had an enchanting butterfly release after our first kiss. On our last day of our time managing Living Waters, we took a walk down by the lake. We saw a butterfly perched on a rock, and it crawled into our hands, as if it were blessing our transition back to Dallas. Butterfly gardens are one of my happy places; my favorite is in Costa Rica where the sky is decorated with large Blue Morpho butterflies.

As I approached the mastectomy, I had secretly made myself a promise that if it were my time to leave this earth as a Bethany, I would return as a butterfly. (And I would definitely play adorable butterfly tricks on people and mess with them.) In an effort to not freak anyone out before my surgery, I had decided to keep this reincarnation plan to myself.

I carried the butterfly and plant outside to my old, vintage wood balcony and sat in meditation. Before I closed my eyes, I noticed a dragonfly had landed on the railing to my right, just under an oak tree.

Holy shit, this is so meant to be. Chills went down my spine. You see, Shelby had also been deeply affected by cancer, having been a caregiver for three of her family members' journeys with cancer. Her son passed away at the age of six. Her stories of his courage and wisdom throughout the process astonished me. She shared with me that there was a point when she was feeling torn about his treatment plan and her son said, "Don't worry Mommy, don't you know the light is in the doctors too? The light is in every-one." This brilliant little six-year-old opened my eyes and heart to a new way of looking at surgery that had completely soothed any remaining nerves. Shelby and her family created the Clayton Dabney Foundation to support children with cancer. After he died, she saw dragonflies appearing in the oddest places, and his family knew in their hearts that Clayton was present.

Remembering this brought tears. I closed my eyes and breathed. I could feel the warmth of the sun on my face. The sound of the wind whistling through the trees. A swell of gratitude overcame me. *Look what I've done. Look what I've been through. It was hard and I did it! I'm still OK! I'm here. Really here.*

I began to gently move my arms, opening and closing them like wings. When I opened my eyes, the butterfly was doing the same. Stretching her wings for the very first time. *Whoa!* The dragonfly continued to just chill and watch as more tears fell from my eyes. I again remembered a deep, purpose-filled connection to this journey and to myself. I got up to go for a walk, and when I returned, my two new friends were gone.

A few days later, I noticed a tight band in my left armpit. It restricted my movement and was incredibly painful, much like a tight piano string running from my armpit down through my forearm and wrist. I showed my plastic surgeon, who encouraged me to keep stretching and massaging it with oil. Believing a gentle approach was always best, I was slow and mindful with this area.

A week later, I met with my breast surgeon, who examined my armpit with concern before announcing that I had developed "axillary web syndrome" or "cording." This is a rare complication that can occur after an axillary lymph node dissection in which scar tissue forms at the surgery site and then long, thick, painful cords form down the arm or chest. Oddly, no one knows for sure what the cords are actually made of—it could be hardening of the lymphatic channels (thus creating a greater risk of lymphedema), blood vessels, or nerves. Its duration is equally mysterious, since cording can last for just a couple of months or a lifetime.

Isn't it funny how once something gets a medical name, it sounds so much scarier? And why does the mind stay obsessed over the word "lifetime" instead of focusing on "a couple of months"?

Although there is little research on what it's made out of, the therapy to address cording is still the same: #stretchand-movethatshit.com.

As the breast surgeon wrote my referral for physical therapy, she explained that I could not begin radiation until I had regained full range of motion on the left side. Since I would need to hold my arms above my head for ten to fifteen minutes during radiation treatments, she wanted me "doing handstands at our next appointment in three weeks." *Geez! No pressure!*

I was also receiving weekly "boob fills" from my plastic surgeon, which made the cording even tighter. This was already a pretty intense process for me, after each fill my chest, rib cage, and shoulder girdle were forced to painfully stretch too. Yet it was also very cool to see my boobs grow half a cup size every week.

After I left the office, my stomach and throat began to tighten. Anger came for a visit. My internal dialogue unfolded something like this: *Are you kidding me? Another damn thing to deal with on top of everything else? I'm just starting to feel "normal" again and now THIS! And why wasn't this band thingy listed in the MASSIVE amount of paperwork I had to read before surgery?!!! I signed off on EVERY possible side effect/complication, including DEATH!!! They didn't prepare me for this!* Then Despair started bargaining: *I just want a break…please. No more universal tests. Enough. White flag is up.* A little whisper from Curiosity snuck in: *Hey, what if this is a good thing? You never know what cool things this could lead to.* Anger plus Despair plus Depression ganged up on Curiosity: *SHUT-UP*

*Ms. Try-to-look-on-the-bright-side-of-everything and just admit
it: this SUCKS BUTT.*

So Anger's gang won for a few hours. And then it was time
to do The Work. Questioning two of the thoughts in particular
really began to shift my experience: *Cording is going to make my
life more difficult. The surgeon didn't prepare me for this complication.*

Through my inquiry, I discovered I had absolutely no proof
that cording would make life more difficult. In fact, I had more
proof that it would make it *easier.* There was nothing "new" I
needed to learn. I had an expert physical therapist for that. Even
though my job as a yoga therapist involved working with bodies
and helping them heal, I had been feeling a little nervous with
my own body after this surgery. So, now my body became my
physical therapist's job! The responsibility was off my shoulders.
In fact, it was quite easy for me. I just had to show up and do what
she said, ask questions, and repeat. It also kept me in my yoga
practice and focused on self-care. *Hmmmm…maybe this cording
thing isn't so bad.*

Through questioning my thoughts about the surgeon, I could
see how well *she did prepare me for this complication.* In fact, the
moment she saw it, she recognized it and sent me directly to
physical therapy. She was also very encouraging about me moving
my arms right after surgery, even while still IN the hospital. I may
have babied my arms too much in fear of injuring myself. So the
thought that *I didn't prepare me for this complication* was truer, and
when I was believing my thoughts, I was full of blame, anger, and
guilt. I saw images of the cords multiplying until I was left with
zero use of my arm for the rest of my life. The thick bands felt so
solid and permanent.

Without these thoughts, I heard a sweet, calm, open-minded
"follow the simple instructions" voice. Anger and despair naturally

fell away, allowing curiosity (our true nature) to step in, joined by an openness to seeing the blessings unfold.

By the time I strolled into my first day of physical therapy, three or four additional cords had joined the fiesta. All I could see was how this was all *for* me. It turned out that physical therapy was super similar to yoga therapy, and it was paid for by insurance. Guess what cording led to? Free private yoga therapy with one of the coolest therapists ever, Tiffany. Her mother was a breast cancer survivor, and Tiffany was a complete expert in this field. I freaking LOVED it! I learned so much about my body, anatomy, alignment, stretching, and strengthening. I even incorporated some of the new moves into my work with my private yoga clients. Yep, cording actually made me better at my job.

As we began our work together, she warned me that the cords could make a crunchy noise and even snap as they broke up. As disturbing as that sounded, apparently it was a good thing. I experienced a small snap at home during self-massage, and then, during one PT session, an extremely loud POP exploded in my armpit as she was stretching me. It was the oddest sensation…like a firework going off in my armpit, but it actually wasn't painful in the moment. The pain came immediately afterwards as I remembered the unfamiliar sound and sensation, leading to an unplanned outburst of, "Holy shit, fuck, shitballz!" in a room full of strangers. I guess you could say I brought my own set of fireworks to PT. *You're welcome. I'm here all week!*

Very quickly, I experienced a drastic shift in my body. I regained my full range of motion along with the confidence to move and use my arms in all of my daily activities. Although the cording was still present, I felt unattached to the outcome, seeing so clearly how I could live a full life with or without this cording. Then, within two months, the cording left me. It vanished just in time for the next phase of treatment: radiation. Future me would have additional visits from my cording friend, and it was still all good. My mind was no longer able to label it as a problem or even a complication, only as a practice of loving what is.

Placing the blame or judgment on someone else leaves you powerless to change your experience; taking responsibility for your beliefs and judgments gives you the power to change them.

—BYRON KATIE

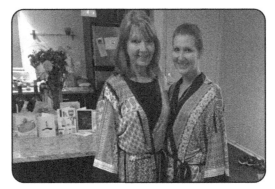

Recovery Robes

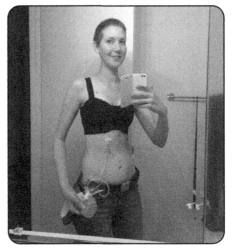

Rocking the Fanny with Drains

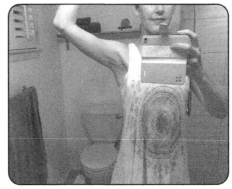

Cording

5 TIPS FOR ROCKING YOUR RECOVERY

1. **Stop trying to be holy and take the drugs, yo.**
   Medicine is a gift, a privilege. If you're in pain, get over your-self and take the meds with gratitude. Still in pain? Ask your doctor if switching meds is right for you.

2. **Question your thoughts about pain.**
   Notice thoughts like *I can't handle this. The pain will get worse. It will last forever.* Is it true? Can you absolutely know it's true? How do you react, what happens, when you believe it? Who would you be without the thought? Now turn it around.

3. **Say YES to help.**
   This is your time to heal, your time to receive. Remember how good it feels to be in service to others. Why would you deny somebody else the gift of helping you? Get specific about what you need: Food? Help getting up? A clean house? A ride?

4. **Connect with your inner child.**
   Ask to be held, snuggled, and petted. See life through a child's eyes—get curious, playful, and silly. Feeling emotional? Throw that tantrum till you're empty.

5. **Notice the blessings and all the things you CAN do.**
   Focus on everything you CAN do. Breathe? Eat? Pee? Walk? Talk? Cry? Watch TV? Read? Sleep? Pause and notice the miracle of the body healing, how supported you are, and what you're learning about yourself. How could it be happening *for* you?

13

Activate the Love Beams: Radiation

BEFORE I DIVE INTO the joy of radiation, we need to have a little chat about life with tissue expander boobs. They had been with me for two months at that point, and dear God…they were completely and totally for my entertainment.

First of all, they needed a different name. As you've probably noticed, re-naming things is a popular coping mechanism of mine. Please choose from the following options: (1) Boobs of Steel, (2) Fembot Tattas, (3) Bowling Ball Boobies, or (4) Bionic Superhero Breasts.

These babies were a true practice of stillness. They did not move. At all. I may have filmed myself in a slow-motion cartwheel to showcase this talent.

After the eight-week filling process, I finally reached my ideal boob size: a small C cup. Because radiation was going to shrink the skin and surrounding tissue, my plastic surgeon blew me up one size bigger on the soon-to-be laser beamed left side. This left me spending the summer of 2016 with a leftie super boob.

When a woman would ask me, "What do they feel like?" I usually immediately grabbed her hand and placed it on my breast. Or I'd offer to go in the bathroom and show her what they looked like. Cancer has a way of instantly dissolving any nakey boundaries; it's just a body, and I was happy to educate anyone about my weird AF boobie situation.

When someone hugged me, they would often ask, "Oh—am I hurting you?" Dude, I was the one with the hardass, indestructible bowling ball boobs that dig into your chest when we hug. "Am *I* hurting *you*?"

I had also learned that they could NOT be used as massage tools. I tried that with my husband, and he wasn't into it. However, they COULD be used to hold a plate of food while watching TV.

Also, I was all over this whole anti-gravity thing. I hadn't realized just how much the weight of my natural breasts had yanked down on my shoulders until the weight was completely lifted. My posture improved, and I rarely got headaches. I gleefully experimented with strappy bras, tank tops, and dresses that I couldn't really wear before.

Still, my chest felt super tight, so, again, daily yoga, massage, and stretching were essential.

I walked into a new wing of the medical center. Through sliding glass doors, a large sign screaming "Danger! Radiation Zone!" greeted me. *What a warm welcome.*

As had become my habit, I went to the appointment by myself. In all honesty, it was also my preference. Mom was in Florida, and Travis wasn't exactly a blast at doctor appointments. He offered to come, but I realized it really wasn't his cup of tea. He had a habit of worrying and asking me a million times if I was OK. "Yes, I'm fine—this is all just part of the process. Can we please have fun with it now?" Or he would whisper in my ear that something the doctor was suggesting wasn't accurate. That was cool if he wanted to believe it, but instead of being the Doctor Devil of Doubt on my right shoulder, maybe HE could find the research, bring it to the doctor, and ask specific questions? Or maybe HE could find me an alternative doctor that HE felt comfortable with? I was open.

I appreciated working with doctors who were physically present with me and could look at my specific body and treat my specific cancer. This also didn't mean that I would just sit back and immediately say "yes" to everything they recommended (although my life might have been easier if I did). I brought tons of questions, I asked to see the research and statistics, I asked about short and long-term side effects, I asked what they would do if they were in my position, I consulted people who had been through it, I looked for complimentary therapies to ease side effects, and I did The Work on my fears. Making peace with cancer doesn't mean you're a doormat. I was extremely engaged and active in my healthcare.

Sometimes I felt Travis was more into bitching about it all than finding an actual alternative solution. Yes, I was annoyed and frustrated with him quite often during that time. It hadn't been easy. And no, I wasn't doing The Work on it. Yet. Very soon, I would learn that I could no longer sweep my frustrations under the rug. But for now, I was focused on laser beams.

"Are there really lasers?" I asked.

"No, not at all." As I shook hands with my radiation oncologist, I couldn't help but giggle as I remembered my breast surgeon's description of him: a tall glass of water. I think we have different tastes in water, but dang—he was tall! And Irish. Not to mention kind and patient with my bazillion questions about the process, statistics, and research. "What's your next question? You get as many as you want."

I learned that the job of radiation was to locally treat the areas where cancer was present and where cancer most commonly recurs. It cleans up microscopic cells that can't be detected in diagnostic scans. In my case, radiation treatment would focus on four main areas: (1) The left breast. (2) The left chest wall. (3) The left axilla. (4) A small pocket of lymph nodes below the left collarbone.

I considered radiation to be the final house cleaning. It could destroy healthy cells as well, but healthy cells can quickly repair themselves. The cancer cells cannot. Of course, as with the rest of the process, there were no guarantees.

"Can I have sex? Or will my vagina be radioactive?" I blurted out. I got such a kick out of asking doctors awkward questions for some reason.

"The moment the machines are turned off, there is no radiation. You are not radioactive in any way, so yes, you can resume all regular routines," he responded, his face professionally expressionless.

After signing more paperwork with long lists of terrifying—wait—*don't know, don't know, don't know* side effects, the one that haunted me the most was "permanent heart condition." My mind latched on, and here we dove again into fear, panic, and my heart nearly jumping out of my chest.

Later, I did The Work on this belief that *radiation will give me a permanent heart condition*. It became evident that my thinking about it was giving me a heart condition right away—why wait for radiation? Also, without the thought, I was free to do more research in peace, ask more questions, and remember the benefits of the treatment.

My heart then found a warm, welcoming home in the Yahoo! Turnaround. *Radiation will give me a permanent heart condition! Yahoo!* Yes, it would give me a heart condition: an open heart. Isn't that what this whole process was all about? Now I had to call it Love Beam Therapy. (Are you sick and tired of my cheesy names yet? Lol. I love them.)

The first day was a simulation. Just as models are fitted for their designer clothing, I was fitted for the radiation table. I walked into a room that looked like a scene from the Matrix. It was actually pretty cool!

Topless, with toe shoes on my feet and a medical muumuu around my hips, I laid down on the table. I was taught the radiation yoga pose of arms over my head with my head slightly tilted to the right. Background music filled my ears with a male rendition of Whitney Houston's "I Will Always Love You." *Romantic.* A sci-fi looking machine slowly danced over me, projecting a graph of red lines over my body for measurements. Tiny blue X's with clear stickers began to fill my torso. I closely resembled a treasure map.

My technician, Tin, was from Asia. He brought with him a dry sense of humor, and I greatly appreciated how meticulous he was with the measurements. I had heard that that was the toughest part of radiation therapy—making sure patients are lined up correctly with the machines so that you don't accidentally give an innocent organ (LIKE MY HEART AND LUNGS) a massive dose of radiation. *Glad it's not my job! I just lie here and breathe.*

After all the "X's" were in place, I got dressed and set up the treatment schedule for the next five-and-a-half weeks. I chose afternoons so I could still teach yoga classes in the mornings. Instead of being annoyed at having a daily cancer treatment appointment (how inconvenient!), I chose to think of it as a new afternoon client…we were doing a six-week love beam series together.

Turns out, radiation was simply a ten-minute meditation. Lie down and assume yoga pose. Relax. Breathe in the belly. Be still. Notice surroundings. Lights. Quiet. Giant machine. In my face. Table moving. Machine circling me. *Is that what's giving me the radiation?* I couldn't tell. I was kinda missing the laser beams that I had imagined. In fact, I couldn't feel anything at all. Close eyes. Back to breathing.

The technician's voice appeared over the speaker, "OK, Bethany—all done."

"Wait. That's it? Are you sure it worked?" I asked in confusion.

"Yeah, it feel like you no get what you pay for."

Alrighty, I'm cool with that. One treatment down, 27 more to go!

FACEBOOK UPDATE

So far, radiation proves to be much scarier in my mind than in reality—the process is actually super easy, quick, and painless. Whew!

After 20 treatments, I do have a lobster sunburn in some areas, and it can be itchy.

Luckily, my mastectomy took away sensory nerves from my breast and armpit so I don't feel any pain. I'm keeping the skin well moisturized, applying concentrated green tea multiple times per day, gooey Aquaphor, and am taking black seed oil pills to decrease side effects.

Some days I'm really tired—all good, I like naps. After each session, I find a spot in nature and lay down for 30 minutes on the earth. Feels like a sweet inner re-balancing. I continue to be amazed at this body and mind.

Also found a surprise in my armpit today. Half of my hair fell out—let freedom ring! Happy Fourth of July everyone!

Towards the end of treatment, I was free-boobing it. Bras were just too irritating to the skin, plus I was seriously gooping on the Aquaphor. It felt like I was constantly covered in beeswax.

As exciting as it was to have boobs that stood up on their own, my nipples did the same. They were a tit bit googly-eyed, especially as the left side continued to get higher and tighter from radiation. My discovery of nipple covers was pretty dang exciting.

One afternoon, I and my newly covered nips went thrift shopping for cheap, loose-fitting shirts that could get gooed up. I already had a new wardrobe of bamboo SPF tops, but I would use any excuse for more retail therapy shopping. While rummaging through tops, I noticed one of my nipple covers was missing. *Crap.*

When did it fall out? And how creepy is it if someone saw a skin-tone colored flap fall out of my shirt? "Excuse me ma'am, is this your nipple?" I retraced my steps through the store, but it was nowhere to be found.

Shopping bags in hand, I walked back to my car, where I found the cover melted into the asphalt by the driver's seat door. Slick as ever, I did an inconspicuous yoga lunge and scooped that baby right up. Problem solved.

July 26th marked the end of my cancer treatment. What an incredible, elated adrenaline high! Yes, I still had more to go with hormone therapy and my final reconstruction surgery, but this was the last big phase for the big C, baby!

Lying down on the radiation table for the last time, I could hardly contain myself. Tears welled up. I breathed through them and remained still so the final treatment could work its magic.

When it was over, the radiation therapist told me, "OK, now you go as far from here as possible." I responded, "I love you, and no offense, I hope to never see you again." We really got each other.

I busted through the doors of the radioactive room and launched into a full-on happy dance, jumping and twirling. *It's done. It's over. Holy shit.*

I headed straight for Travis and wrapped my arms around him. We had a celebratory make-out session, and I was delighted by his squirmy discomfort from knowing the staff was watching. I loved holding onto that kiss just a little too long, just like our wedding day.

The staff then surprised me with my own personal bell to ring, a plaque, and a homemade cancer survivor graduation hat. Before my last treatment, I had asked if the staff did anything special for patients ending radiation, and they had said "no." They had gone out of their way and created all of this for me. Which of course made me cry even more. I was blown away with gratitude.

As I stood in the long, quiet white hallway waiting for my discharge appointment with the nurse, I held onto Travis and kept crying. I was so fucking happy. I couldn't believe it.

The next day, my plastic surgeon filled my right boob to match my left super boob. Then, after my breast surgeon appointment, I heard the cancer patient's dream words: "See you in three months."

Holy moly, this new reality of no more weekly (sometimes daily) doctor visits, no more big treatments, was starting to settle in. I had to take this sweet body on a celebratory month-long vacation with my favorite travel buddy: ME!

As the plane lifted off from DFW, my eyes began to water again. I was now just a regular gal living an amazingly free-flowing life. Yes, I still had fembot boobs and was wearing an arm condom to prevent lymphedema, but I had hair now. I didn't look cancery at all! My curls were even coming back! The first one started as a flip underneath my left ear and grew into a plump sausage curl. I named him Fred.

The trip kicked off with a few days in NYC with my sister-in-law, Annie, and we joined our soon-to-be sister-in-law, Emma, for her bachelorette party in Brooklyn. We drank wine, ate great food, and danced until 3:00 am. It felt like I was channeling my time in Spain all over again. Impressively, this body was keeping up with the younger girls. I loved the shocked look on their faces when they heard I had just finished cancer treatment.

Proudly, I lifted up my shirt to show them my amazing new breasts and was met with frozen faces of horror. *Hey, I thought they looked pretty good?* I mean, yeah, sure the skin on the radiation side was peeling off and my boob was being pulled up to my collarbone…but it wasn't the "mutilated, barbaric" picture I had heard about. *Or is it? Is that what they're thinking?* I called myself out: *Hey I'm trying to live out of their heads. I have no idea what they're thinking, and to be honest, how I feel about myself is more important. Back to staying in my business.*

One sunny blue-sky day, we ate lunch at Smorgasburg, an outdoor flea market of around 100 eclectic food tents. Standing in line for some vegetarian Venetian wrappy things, I asked the woman in front of me if she would take my picture. She inquired what brought me to Brooklyn, so I told her that I was here for a bachelorette party, then blurted out, "I also just finished a year of cancer treatment!" She exclaimed, "Oh my God—ME TOO!" She had recently had her final reconstruction surgery and asked if I wanted to feel her breasts. *Ummm…yes, please!* Within seconds of meeting, I was feeling up a stranger's boobs in public. *Wow, they feel so soft and natural.*

After the high energy of NYC, I boarded a train to Westpoint to stay with my girlfriend, Krissy, and her cute-as-a-button baby girl. We had known each other since third grade and had so much fun lounging around, cooking meals, and reminiscing about all of the crazy things we used to do when we were "young." Like ODing on Pixie Sticks (*is that how I got cancer?*), playing "spot the mullet" at monster truck rallies, and singing Reba McEntire in empty parking lots. Now we had grown up into such mature women… *right.* Time is a funny concept, isn't it?

I hopped back on a train to Boston, where I stayed with my younger brother, Jordan, Emma, and my furry niece. We spent our days walking, doing yoga, and eating yet more amazing food. Since I was now more "flexitarian" in my diet, I treated myself to local fresh breads, organic coffee, wine, and some kickass chocolate desserts. And oh, yes, real pizza…how I've missed you. Overall, my energy was definitely coming back, but I still needed an afternoon siesta to make it through the day.

With a full belly and fuller heart, I boarded a bus to Burlington, VT, to visit my friend from The Work, Todd, and his partner. I devoured their homemade Ayurvedic meals. When night fell, we swam in the crystal-clear water of Lake Champlain under the full moon. It felt cleansing and purifying. It sounds crazy, but I was literally living on a high of gratitude.

The next day, I moved into the finale of my sabbatical: a weeklong *Love is the Power* retreat led by Tom Compton in the countryside of Abercorn, Quebec. A rustic, cozy four-bedroom farmhouse nestled in the colorful rolling hills, gardens, and forest provided the perfect backdrop for dropping into inner work. Two of my sweetest friends from The Work, Sarah Maya and Susan, were hosting the event and had invited me to join free of charge as a post-treatment gift. #peoplearesokind

In such a loving and supportive environment, I was free to explore deep fears around cancer returning, self-judgments about choosing conventional medicine, the fear of death, and much more.

Vegetarian meals, walking meditation, dancing like no one's watching…and I even led a few morning yoga classes outside. It was the perfect experience for my mind, body, and soul. One key takeaway I was continuing to explore was *Who would I be without the label of "right" and "wrong"*? What a fascinating question! I noticed that so much of my life was lived out of needing to know "the right way" and "the right answers." *What if it's ALL right? ALL good? ALL love? God, wouldn't that be a relief?*

After the retreat, Susan and I spent a few nights in the beautiful city of Montreal before my flight home. I loved hearing French every day and was already plotting my return. Although I experienced sadness ending such an epic trip, I was also excited to return to my "new" life in Dallas.

I began taking tamoxifen, a drug used to prevent the recurrence of estrogen-positive cancers. It is a systemic treatment (meaning it treats the whole body), and if there are any remaining cancer cells, it will bind their mouths closed so that they cannot feed on estrogen. No food = no life.

You may have guessed that I had mixed feelings about taking any type of drug for five to ten years, and I did my best to explore a well-researched alternative. Each doctor and naturopath I consulted with had the same answer: there was no alternative. Because I was young and knew this body was awesome at producing estrogen (a.k.a. "cancer candy"), it was very important to me to address this part of the cancer treatment plan. The way I saw it, tamoxifen was the best option available for me at that moment, and I was also open to that changing.

My oncologist put it nicely: "I don't like to tell anyone that they will be taking a drug for ten years…because we don't know. New research could show up or circumstances may change. Let's just try it out and see how you do." When I picked up the bottle from the pharmacy, I laughed out loud when I saw the tiny, innocent tablet that resembled a baby aspirin. I had been picturing some kind of huge, scary horse pill with spikes on it. No crazy side effects appeared other than getting a little hot flashy at night, and it was also summer in Texas, so who didn't?

A new chapter in life had definitely begun. The universe was already giving me some really cool opportunities! I was invited to create yoga videos for CanSurround™, a web-based tool designed to help patients with the mental and emotional journey through cancer. I had met the founders at a Byron Katie conference and knew we were meant to work together. I had so much fun creating the videos with my own cancer adventures in mind, and I hoped they would support others in moving through their experiences with more grace and ease.

Incredibly, I was seeing my work shift into helping others find peace around pain and illness. My new private clients were cancer thrivers or facing other health challenges. I partnered with my friend, Helena, to lead an online *Making Peace with Disease* class series. Through her own experience with HIV, Helena had also found an indescribable state of freedom using The Work of Byron Katie. As I witnessed her presentation at the same Byron Katie conference, I was moved to tears realizing how we all go through similar mental journeys when it comes to dis-ease. Even though the conditions may be very different, the root of our stress is the same: believing our thoughts.

Along these lines, I led my first workshop as part of a breast cancer retreat at my local cancer support center. About thirty women of all ages and backgrounds gathered there, with one common thread: cancer. As I introduced the process of The Work and shared my experience, together we worked through one of our universal cancer thoughts: *I need to be strong.*

Through the four questions, we could see how much pressure we put on ourselves to be perfect, to hold in our pain, and act like everything's great. Without the thought, there is permission to love ourselves, just as we are. Permission to grieve, be vulnerable, rest, and ask for help.

In the turnarounds, one young woman wearing a floral scarf wrapped around her head raised her hand from the back of the room and shared an example of how *I don't need to be strong* is truer. She had a blended family, and before her diagnosis, she felt a separation from her stepchildren. They just weren't connecting. It wasn't until she broke down in front of them in the middle of treatment that they finally saw her as human and let her in. They had never been closer. Yeah, there weren't a lot of dry eyes in that room!

We also looked at *I need to be weak* and noticed that weakness is nothing more than a false label, a story. Is it really weak to practice self-care, slow down, and rest? Doesn't it take true strength to break down and be vulnerable? These women were amazing. I felt so connected to them and so meant to be there. I would never have been able to experience any of this if it wasn't for my Guru Cancer.

On September 4th, I celebrated my 35th birthday. I sensed that birthdays would officially take on a brand-new meaning now that I was just so grateful to have each one! I get to get older! Aging is a privilege, yo.

One year earlier, if someone would have told me, "Guess what?!! Those lulu lumps in your boobies and armpit are CANCER and in ONE year, you will have been through five months of chemo, lost your mermaid hair, had your natural breasts surgically removed and replaced with boobs-of-steel tissue expanders, and floated through five-and-a-half weeks of radiation therapy," I would have responded, "YOU CRAZY." And then if you said, "And even more surprising is that you will actually ENJOY a lot of it. It will open your heart in ways you never thought possible. It will open doors that you never knew existed.

It will give you strength, purpose, presence, and gratitude. You will feel an enormous amount of love and support from so many. It will be one of the greatest gifts of your life." I would have said, "WHAT? NOW YOU REALLY CRAY CRAY."

As this new, exciting chapter of my life was unfolding, a painful voice inside of me began to get louder and louder. I couldn't ignore it anymore. I finally gave myself space to listen to it. Its name was Rage, and it was heading directly for Travis.

The teacher you need is the person you're living with.

—BYRON KATIE

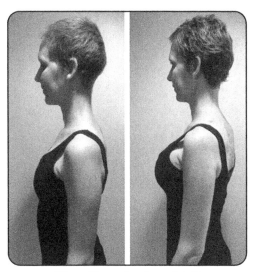

Tissue Expanders from A to D

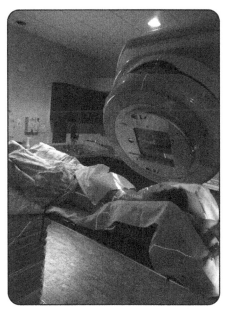

Love Beam Therapy

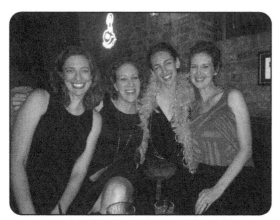

Bachelorette Party in NYC

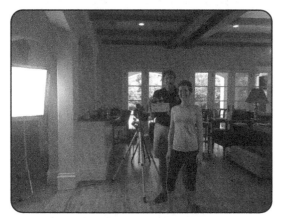

Filming Yoga Videos for CanSurround

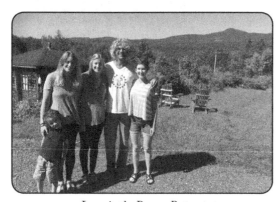

Love is the Power Retreat

14

The Perfect Cancer Husband

I HAD THE PERFECT CANCER HUSBAND, always loving, calm, and understanding. He told me everything was going to be OK and that he was here for me and supported me no matter what. When I was in doubt, he would tell me I was making all of the right decisions. He thought I was sexy as hell, even when I was bald and looked like a little alien. When things were tough, he could always lift my spirits; he made even the most challenging times fun, lighthearted, and exciting. He loved and trusted me unconditionally. I could always count on him.

Yes, I did have the perfect cancer husband. There was just one problem: he lived in my head. He was a figment of my imagination—a fantasy. And as I continued to hold that perfect husband image in my mind, my real husband didn't stand a chance. He fell short. Every. Time.

Travis and I were not in a good place. We hadn't been for some time, and I had been afraid to admit it to myself. Sometimes he was amazing, but more often I wanted to strangle him. We argued so much. Our sex life disappeared. I honestly had more fun without him. So why be married? I was beginning to see divorce as the only inevitable outcome. *Wow, I might actually be going from the Big C right into the Big D.*

Remember how magical my marriage was when I was first diagnosed? It was as if we couldn't waste one single moment together; life was too precious. I instantly saw how cancer could be the most incredible bonding experience between us, a glue that could make our marriage even stronger. As our relationship started going downhill, it felt like a rude slap in the face. Here I was experiencing all of these amazing blessings with cancer, yet it was completely fucking up my marriage.

How could two people with such different perspectives on healing live in the same house? How could I be at peace with my treatment plan when the person I loved the most didn't agree with it? And if it was actually possible that I might not have as much time on this earth as I thought, wouldn't I want to spend it with someone who could really enjoy it with me? I was so tired of being the driver of fun and joy in our relationship. The one who made tough times better. I felt so alone. Where did my partner go?

It seemed like any time I brought up good news or found something to be excited about, Travis found a way to poo all over it. For example:

Me: "Look honey, I think I'm finally gaining some weight back!"

Him: "Ummmm...really? I don't see it."

Me: "How sweet! Robyn made me this awesome body scrub from essential oils!"

Him: "There's sugar in it! Sugar feeds cancer."

Me: "Guess what?! My period is gone! Yeah!!!"

Him: "Oh my God…What is this chemo doing to your body?"

At first, the fact that he wouldn't get help from others drove me insane. *He needs more support* was constantly running through my mind. Now this desire may appear to have come from a loving wife, but to be totally honest, it was 100% selfish. I wanted him to get support so I could feel better about myself and my decisions. I wanted him to have fun and be happy so I could be free to do the same. Co-dependency at its finest. *But I'm justified—I'm the one with cancer after all!*

During one of my 2:00 am writing sprees, I decided to write a letter to myself as if it were written by my husband. I included all of the things I wished he would say and do for me, how he could make the perfect cancer husband a reality.

A Letter from My Husband (written by Me)

Dear Bethany,

Honey, how do you feel about all of this right now? You are free to tell me anything and I will listen with an open, non-judgmental heart. I want you to know I think you are beautiful and sexy no matter what. You can't make a wrong decision—whichever path you choose, it is the right one and we'll get through it together. I will always back you 100%.

I am so sorry about being so intense with you in the past. I've been an asshole. I understand that voicing my opinions so loudly has put you in a difficult place between me and the doctors. It has nothing to do with you—this is my own shit—and I am going to stop trying to control your treatment. I'll be your loving husband, not your doctor. If I'm stressed, I'll take it to inquiry and find my own freedom.

I see the reality that so far the treatment plan is working! You are handling it all perfectly. Let's cherish each moment we have together and live a fun, exciting life full of adventures. I love you with all of my heart.

Love,
Travis

As I quietly imagined hearing these words from him, it felt so comforting. I could really see him genuinely feeling this way in his heart. In fact, he had actually said many of these things to me before. *Why does my mind latch on only to the negative? Maybe his ego was just getting in the way of always showing up in a loving way. What if he is innocent?*

Then I re-read the same letter as if it was written by me to myself. *Oh wow, this was all so fucking true. I've been so here for me.* But when I was consumed with what he should feel, say, think, and do, I would totally leave that sweet place with myself. If I lived out this letter to myself and really believed it, I could be at peace regardless of how my hubby behaved. This felt so empowering.

I read the letter again, this time as if I had written it to him. *Whoa.* This hit me differently. It was also true. I *could* be there for him. *Wait a minute, I've been such an asshole to him! I've been short, impatient, and not compassionate. I've been so wrapped up in my own issues and rarely took the time to put myself in his shoes and consider just how hard all of this is for him. Then there're my crazy lady mood swings where I've gone totally off on him. God, it kills me to treat him this way. It hurts so much. What if I could always listen to him with an open heart?* Now I could see that he was also making amazing decisions—one of which was to stay with me even though he thought the treatment would kill me. That took courage and strength.

Byron Katie often says that if you think someone else needs The Work, then *you* need to do The Work. It's projection. So I *finally* started questioning more beliefs, beliefs like *I need him to agree with my treatment plan. He isn't supporting me. I can't count on him. He is ruining my peace in cancer treatment.*

This got me through treatment with more peace. I became more aware of the ways my husband helped me on a daily basis. He made me organic green juices *every* morning, he worked seven days a week to financially support me when I needed time off, and he held me when I was crying. He did offer to go with me to appointments or give me rides. He did The Work with me. He told me on so many occasions that I was courageous.

While these realizations had been enlightening and connecting, I had also been doing The Work with a motive. A motive to avoid feeling the deep, underlying painful emotions.

What's so ingenious about bodies is that they don't let you get away with shit. The migraines came back full force. I could feel a slow build up of resentment circulating throughout my body. Dear God, I honestly couldn't take it anymore. Now that the big phases of treatment were over, it nailed me like a ton of bricks: I was in full husband PTSD.

Over New Year's, I attended Byron Katie's *Mental Cleanse* in Los Angeles, followed by The Institute for The Work's Annual Convention. I wanted the time away to sort out my feelings. After the events, I sat in the hotel lobby with some girlfriends, one of whom was Roxann, Byron Katie's daughter.

Roxann had been leading workshops called *Sitting in the Fire,* which is a unique experience of The Work that combines inquiry "from the early days" and some circle work. It is a way to really delve into Question 3—*how you react, what happens when you're believing a painful thought*—and to let all of the emotions fully express themselves until you're completely empty. This expression can take the form of anything from curling up into a ball and quietly whimpering, screaming at the top of your lungs, to aggressively hitting pads with a plastic bat. It's ALL welcome. She and everyone in the circle holds you in a safe, non-judgmental space throughout the entire process.

I witnessed a sample of this workshop at the convention. The participant in the circle was working on a stressful situation entirely different from my own, yet I felt her grief and rage. Or rather, witnessing her intense emotions gave me permission to get in touch with my own. When it ended, I couldn't get out of that room fast enough.

As soon as the green light appeared on the keypad to my hotel room, I busted through the creaky door. A waft of laundry detergent and bleach filled my nose as my eyes quickly scanned the room to make sure my roommate wasn't there. *Thank God I'm alone.* I face-planted onto the bed of freshly pressed linens and lit my own fire. Screaming into the pillows, I flailed around on the bed like an uncontrollable fish out of water. I hit the mattress again and again until my arms turned into loose spaghetti. It was the physical expression of these words: "F you Travis! F you for not being there for me!" And it was just the beginning.

Chilling in the lobby on an oval couch at the base of the escalator, the girls and I were sipping on coffees and chatting up a storm. Roxann asked, "Should we go back to the hotel room and do a *Sit in the Fire* together?" *Gulp.* The anticipation of being exposed carved a pit in my stomach as the six of us rode the elevator up to the 10th floor. We formed a circle around the two queen beds, with plenty of pillows surrounding us. Roxann invited us to begin by checking in with our emotions. When we felt moved to do so, we shared, saying "I'm in touch with _____ emotion. And with that, I'm in." As it got closer to my turn, my heart jumped into my throat. I could barely breathe, and I was choking back tears. Before I knew it, I heard myself say, "I'm in touch with sadness, disappointment…and fucking rage towards my husband" and began to sob. The circle of women organically shifted towards me, moving in closer, like a pack of mamma wolves who protect their cub. *Uh oh…Looks like I'm the one going into the fire.*

Roxann invited me to choose someone in the circle who represented Travis, someone who carried a similar trait or energy that reminded me of him. I chose my friend, Jodi, who had similar hair. I also knew she was tough as hell and could handle my wild, untamed emotions.

And that's exactly what came out; it was like a volcano erupting inside of me. I pled, begged, yelled, screamed. They banded together to form a wall of pillows so I could safely yet aggressively push against it with all of my force. This energy moving through me was unstoppable. Roxann caught the most painful belief that unconsciously spewed out of my mouth, "Travis, you're the worst part of cancer treatment." *Ouch.* It stabbed my heart. As she repeated my words back to me, shame and guilt hit hard. *How could I think this way about my husband? What kind of person does that?* Roxann asked, "What's the sound?"

A cry of raging desperation sprung out from my throat into a pillow, accompanied by a pool of slobber and snot. I was sure security would be knocking on the door at any moment.

"How does this thought color your world?" Roxann was fiercely and compassionately connected to me. Tears were falling from the other women's eyes.

And oh my God—I could see so clearly how my mind was completely laser focused on every single thing Travis did wrong. It was endless. And it hurt me so much to hate him. I had become totally blind to everything he was doing right, which was a lot! I had also been blind to how hard this process had been for him. *Jesus, look at his past!* His father left when he was little and had never been a part of his life. His first serious girlfriend, his very first true love, died in a drunk driving accident his freshman year in college. He held her hand in the hospital bed, looking into her deformed and swollen face. She was already pronounced brain dead, yet he watched tears fall from her eyes as he said his final goodbyes.

Just two years later, his amazing saint of a grandmother, who was like a mother to him, died of a sudden heart attack. He was completely crushed. This man had been through so much loss. And then the love of his life got cancer? *Oh my God, how did I not see all of this before?* His reactions and struggles made so much sense now. No wonder this was all hitting him harder than I thought it would; no wonder he was trying to control things—he didn't want to lose me too. *Gosh, he is so allowed, so entitled, to go through his process of what's happening to his wife.* Just because I had cancer, I didn't own the exclusive rights to suffering.

Without my stressful stories about him, I was now free to listen to his pain. Free to walk in his shoes. It was complete compassion. Like Jodi was for me in this circle, I could be his placeholder for him to truly express how he felt. It wasn't personal. And it was intimate. So intimate. Wasn't this what I wanted in my marriage? Full, vulnerable, uncensored honesty? Wow, could this actually be possible with him?

After what felt like hours of emptying out my insides, I became aware of the time. My flight was leaving in an hour and a half. As I said my heartfelt thank you's and goodbyes to my circle of women, life felt lighter…like floating in slow motion. It was a high without the drugs! The universe quite literally cleared the way for me to make my flight on time; there was zero traffic during rush hour, I walked right up to the security line, and I even had time to grab a piece of vegan chocolate cake before I boarded the plane. *Hell ya!*

As I sat on the plane, I watched a funny chick flick and devoured my chocolate cake. It was the perfect date with myself, thousands of miles up in the air and completely at home in my heart.

I chose not to tell Travis about this experience. I kept it for me. And I chose to live out my realizations with him instead.

Cancer can definitely be a catalyst that strengthens romantic relationships, but it doesn't always work out that way. I think cancer or any huge life event has a way of highlighting any pre-existing conditions or challenges in relationships. My need for Travis's love and approval for how I live my life existed before cancer. In fact, remember the war I had with my parents? Well, turns out I had unknowingly transferred the same approval-seeking party right over to my husband. Cancer had brought it all to the surface so that it could be exposed, understood, and healed. This was an opportunity to love without conditions and to step into my own power and truth.

One week before my final reconstruction surgery, I co-led an *Inner Peace Retreat* with my dear friend, Susan. We were nestled in the Austin Hill Country at our old stomping grounds, Living Waters…the fairy-tale space where Travis and I were married, where we created a business together, where I did the deep inner work in the certification program that prepared me for meeting cancer with an open mind.

Joined by fourteen participants including my husband, the weekend creatively combined yoga, The Work, meditation, vegetarian meals, and heartfelt community. I was in for a big surprise.

On the last day of the retreat, we invited participants to bring to mind what they were most ashamed of in their life and to identify the painful thoughts underlying that shame.

This is a very raw exercise that gives you the time to sit with the uncomfortable, terrifying, shameful things that we think make us who we are. Moreover, we think we're the only ones carrying this crappy baggage. It isn't just about identifying the shame; it's an (optional) opportunity to stand up amongst a group of people who were strangers less than 36 hours ago, look into their eyes, and expose your damaged goods.

Sounds fun, eh? Where do I sign up, you ask?

It is one of the most intimate practices in The Work, and one of its gifts is that you get to see that everyone else is just like you. We've all done things we are not proud of. We all hold onto secrets that create shame, separation, and loneliness. I like to tell people, "You're not special. We all have the same BS (Belief Systems) floating around in our heads."

But we get really good at hiding. Really good at pretending ourselves into self-love. And just when we start to feel good about ourselves—when we think, "Hey! I'm kinda rocking this thing called Life"—we get nailed by the mean inner voice gnawing at our cover story: "Remember this? You suck!!!" *Ahhhh…the ego.*

As we dove into the exercise, we watched participants one by one share their most ashamed beliefs. We were all in tears. Their vulnerability moved me. I related to each and every one. Susan asked, "Does anyone else feel moved to share?" Before my logical mind could intercept, I heard the voice inside my body say, "I do."

So I stood up and shared my deepest shame—the belief nagging at me as I came to the end of treatment. The one that had created a shameful barrier between me and my husband.

What I felt most ashamed of was that *I couldn't trust alternative medicine to heal me.* And what did that mean about me? What had I been carrying around with me since I started conventional, Western treatment?

It meant that *I am a fraud. I shouldn't work in the wellness industry. I'm not spiritual enough. I will be punished with a lifetime of side effects. People judge me. I did it wrong.* And what hurt the most was the thought that *my husband is completely disappointed in me.*

Slowly, I made eye contact with each participant, feeling seen, heard, and understood, but still scared shitless. Then I met my husband's eyes. Tears of remorse welled up…"I am so sorry! I just couldn't do it!" I cried. He had tears in his eyes too. Tears of love and understanding.

This may sound like nothing to you. People get disappointed in life, right? Not everyone is going to agree with our actions and words. Especially partners. While anger had been telling me that he let me down, this exercise opened up a secret well of shameful beliefs: *I let him down. And I let myself down. I wasn't totally at peace with my choice of treatment.*

I had pretended to be strong, to be confident. I had pretended to be in full acceptance of the medical world. This was my cover story. But I didn't always feel at peace.

After I shared my list, I felt my body shaking and trembling. Then Susan (oh Susan and her laser-like vision into making sure your shit is all cleared up) asked me, "Are you open to taking this further?"

Again, the voice in my body responded before the ego could interrupt. "Yes." And ego jumped in with, "But I notice the thought that retreat leaders aren't supposed to be the one's doing this. The attention should be on the participants."

Susan replied with a smile and shrugged, "Too bad. Now lay on the floor." *OK, we're doing this.* As I laid down, she invited the participants to form a circle around me and, with my permission, to place their hands on me. The effect was one of every inch of me being cradled. Before I knew it, my body was in an earthquake, almost a Tourette's syndrome-style shaking and contorting. I began to wail.

I cried for the me that was scared, ashamed, and confused. I cried for the months of stored-up anger at Travis. I cried for each uncomfortable conversation defending treatment. Honestly, I didn't know what else I was sobbing for, yet I felt so safe and nurtured to let it (whatever "it" was) release through me. *Oh my god, this feeling is incredible.*

My eyes closed, I could feel a sea of hands touching me without a clue about which hands belonged to which body. It didn't matter. Two were massaging my head and neck, and I was being touched like a small child, held and cradled. A voice arose in me: *Bethany, you don't deserve this love. It isn't fair to the others. You are so selfish.* Immediately, the voice was met with "Is it true? Whose business am I in? How do I know this isn't exactly what I need? What everyone here needs?" *Screw it. I'm in.*

It felt like hours of rocking in this ocean of unconditional love and support, when in reality it was only minutes. "This… Is… So… Fucking… Sweet…" I murmured between sobs. I heard laughter and tears.

The yoga pose I was lying in, known as savasana or corpse pose, was very fitting. Part of me died on that stone floor. The part of me that was embarrassed by treatment. The part of me that felt rage and regret towards my husband. The part of me that was scared of being seen as less than perfect. I was finally free to move on.

The hands moved away from my body, and as I sat up, I opened my eyes, asking, "Where's Travis?" I reached for my husband whose hands had been there the whole time. Not just in the circle, but by my side throughout everything, even though his mind might have gotten in the way of being present and supportive the way I would've preferred. The way he would've also preferred. We had that in common.

The group split up into pairs, and I went off with my husband to do inquiry on these underlying beliefs. I humbly learned that *I was wrong*. Although it was hard at first, he had accepted my treatment plan and eventually agreed that it was the best choice for me. He wasn't disappointed in me; in fact, he was actually the opposite: proud. As we talked, Travis admitted how harshly he judged himself for how he treated me and how regretful he felt. He even concurred that the evidence for the effectiveness of alternative medicine wasn't yet sufficient to abandon conventional treatment. And deep down, he was absolutely terrified of losing me.

Travis explained that he wanted to take my pain away. His masculine need to "take control" and "fix things" couldn't be expressed, leaving him feeling helpless. I had also made all of these huge treatment decisions without him, decisions that affected both of our lives. At first, he channeled it all into work with an overwhelming sense of responsibility to save enough money in case we needed to fly off to Mexico to save my life (which, in a way, turned out to be true).

After months of struggling, he finally took his own stress to inquiry. It wasn't until he had made peace with his worst fear, my death, that he was finally able to let go and surrender. He loved me that much. Deep down, his actions were love disguised as fear.

It's hard for me to explain it in words, but something in me shifted. Something cleared in me that allowed me to really see, really feel the innocence of myself and Travis. If I had to give it a label, I'd call it *forgiveness*.

Is there really anything to forgive? We both did the best we could given what we were thinking and believing. We had admitted to each other when we were off and apologized. *So what's the point of holding onto this pain, blame, and shame?* There was NO point. It hurt so badly. It didn't serve anyone. It was a prison. And it was finally ready to let go of me.

My Guru Cancer. My Guru Husband. When I'm open to it, everything in life is my teacher. In this case, they were teaching me the courage of being completely raw and vulnerable. They were teaching me how to totally let go and surrender, how to fall into trust with myself. How to love in disagreement. To have fearless, open communication. To move forward with compassion while honoring the pain and suffering. To see that what lay underneath the reactions, the fear, the terror, the helplessness was nothing more than misguided, innocent *love*. With all of this self-growth and mind-blowing epiphanies, perhaps I really did have the perfect cancer husband after all.

The timing couldn't have been more perfect. My final reconstruction surgery was scheduled for that week.

Once we begin to question our thoughts, our partners, alive, dead, or divorced, are always our greatest teachers. There is no mistake about the person you're with; he or she is the perfect teacher for you, whether or not the relationship works out, and once you enter inquiry, you come to see that clearly. There's never a mistake in the universe.

—BYRON KATIE

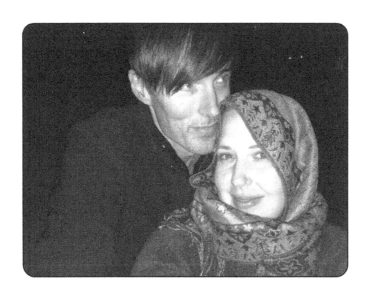

15

Land of BFE

GUESS WHO WAS GETTING NEW BOOBS? This girl.

The day before was filled with adrenaline holy-shit excitement combined with a serious dose of confusing, yet liberating, crying. After almost two years of cancer treatment, the finale was just around the corner. *It's really happening. I actually did this.* I wrapped my arms around myself for a soothing self hug. *So proud of me!*

The spirit of a 13-year-old boy had also been taking over, leaving me seriously breast-obsessed. It was all I could think about. Boobs, boobs, boobs—everywhere I went. I analyzed other women's shape, size, how their breasts bounced and moved, wondering what they felt like. Boobs were just so cool.

I created a folder on my computer's desktop titled "Boobs We Like," and over the months, Travis and I had way too much fun filling it with an array of sexy photos. See? We also had some fun with cancer. How easily the mind forgets. This totally normal relationship bonding exercise does come with some warnings, such as when you type "breast" in Google, be prepared for some disturbing images. I wanted to see nice, pretty, simple boobs. Preferably not ones in the midst of an orgy being covered by giant penises. (P.S. NEVER Google "mastectomy" unless you want to be met with every worse-case scenario image your mind could have ever imagined. Oh crap, I probably just made you curious. You're on Google right now, aren't you? Don't do it!!!)

Geesh this adrenaline is insane. *Is it time yet? Can I get new boobs now?* My thinking is also anxious: *How will they look? How will they feel? Will I like them? What if something goes wrong? That was a lot of potential "complications" I signed off on. Again. Oh wait— don't know, don't know, don't know. Deep breaths.*

A few weeks ago, Travis and I brought our sexy boob photos to the plastic surgeon so we could all plan the details of my future breasts in the pre-op visit. Three souls joining together to create the ultimate masterpiece. I was giddy with excitement.

It was quite possible that I was his first patient to be so "prepared." *How is this not a thing?* As the surgeon sorted through the photos, I was surprised that he seemed impatient and irritated.

He told us, "They won't look like this because you don't have breasts. I don't know what to tell you—what you have aren't breasts." *WTF.* A surge of defense and anger arose in me. I swallowed back tears. *How dare you say I don't have breasts! Yes, I do! Just 'cuz they are expanders or implants doesn't mean they aren't breasts! You should NEVER say this to a woman in cancer treatment. And this is the man who I am trusting my body with? Where is his compassion? Screw you!* Inside, a war was brewing, yet on the outside, I was silently witnessing the activity. *Hold on sweet mind of mine, what do I really want in this situation?*

I want the surgeon to be kind to me. I caught the thought in the heat of the moment. That is another cool side effect of an ongoing practice of inquiry—you get better at capturing the thoughts *before* going into full reaction mode. As the surgeon stepped out so I could get undressed for the examination, I looked to Travis for comfort. Tears welled up in my eyes, like a little girl who had just been told Santa isn't real…by a big mean boob bully. Travis offered, "Maybe he's just having a bad day and it's not personal."

I took in his words. It could be true—doctors are human too. How often do we forget this? They get into arguments with their spouses, their bodies are overworked and tired, they have difficult patients, and for all I know, someone could have unexpectedly died on his table that very morning. I couldn't know his mind, his world. Whatever was going on, he just didn't seem like his usual, upbeat self. Maybe this wasn't the real him.

My mind jumped to the turnaround: *I want me to be kind to him.* And then I realized that maybe my hot model photos were putting just a lil' too much pressure on him to create the perfect breasts. Maybe he was worried that my expectations were too high and that he'd disappoint me. In my mind, I want to be kind to him too—it doesn't feel good inside of me to see him as the Big Boobie Bully A-hole.

As he walked back into the room, I apologized to him for possibly coming off as high maintenance. I assured him that I was the type of person who could find happiness in anything and not to worry. Immediately his entire demeanor shifted as he apologized to me for coming off as curt, saying that he just wanted me to be happy with the results and that he would do the best he could. Working with radiated tissue can be unpredictable, and while he would do everything in his power to achieve a good cosmetic outcome, it doesn't always work out that way. I now heard him as trying to inform me and educate me, and I appreciated this.

I want me to be kind to me. It was important for me to hold my truth that I did have breasts, they were simply now made of a material that was less likely to get cancer. I told myself to breathe, relax, and remember that everyone here was supporting me on the final leg of this trip. I told myself that I was beautiful, no matter what. I remembered Nainoa's words, "You're still the same person," regardless of what my body looked like.

We then dove into the details of the procedure, including the type, size, and projection of my implants. I had opted to go with his recommendation of the newest round "gummy bear" implant that felt the most natural, was leak-proof, and had the longest life, up to 30 years. Originally, saline had sounded like the best option until I realized that the outer shell was the same material as a gummy implant. In addition, if you spring a leak—which can happen anytime, anywhere—your boob basically deflates and you'll need another surgery. Saline implants had to be replaced approximately every 10 years. Dammit, here I was again, changing my mind to choose the "less natural" option. Yet it was what felt best for me. I loved the thought of a future with fewer surgeries.

The surgeon plopped the gummy implant into my hand. I squished it around, put it under my shirt to cop a feel, and tossed it up and down before handing it over to Travis for a few squeezes too. How strange that these would soon live inside of me.

When I first met with my plastic surgeon over a year ago, he had handed me a pamphlet of his work, and I remembered one woman in particular who stood out: *Samantha. Samantha's boobs are amazing. Give me Samantha's boobs. Yes, please.* Remember how Samantha was also the name of my alter ego when I wore my sexy wig during chemo? *Could this be destiny? I think so.*

The surgeon said that my implants would be similar to hers,

commenting that she was actually now a bikini model. New career in my future?

His assistant walked us through how the surgery would work. It was much shorter than my previous one (about 2 hours), and the recovery was supposed to be much easier. He would enter through the scars from the mastectomy, make smaller incisions, and replace the tissue expanders (SEE YA and won't miss ya AT ALL) with the implants.

What was super weird was that while I was off in a deep, drug-induced sleep, he would strap me down, prop me upright on the operating table, and try on about five different implant sizes to see which one looked best. *Eeeek!* Yet I also so appreciated that they do this! Boobs look very different when lying down versus sitting up. I asked if Travis could come in and give the final OK, but apparently that could be a very traumatic experience for him. *OK, I get it, perhaps he's already been through enough trauma!*

After all that fun, the surgeon would then liposuction fat from my love handles and put it into my breasts for extra padding between the implant and skin and to help to shape the breasts. I had been a good girl, diligently working very hard on building this fat with the help of nightly chocolate peanut butter Coconut Bliss ice cream. It was a rough job, but somebody had to do it (#cancerbonus). With hard work, I had gained 15 pounds back from my lowest weight in chemo, and it was so fun to see and feel my curves again. So to be clear, I would soon be wearing my Coconut Bliss muffin tops in my breasts. *This is crazy.* And even crazier was that very soon I would be someone who could say that I had had a boob job and lipo. *How very Dallas of me!*

I tried not to think about the procedure details too much since they creeped me out. Actually, it was my thoughts that were creeping me out—the procedure didn't even exist yet outside of my head. It definitely takes a certain type of person to stomach this work, and I was grateful for the expertise of my surgeon and his staff. That was not a job I could handle. All I had to do was show up, go to sleep, and wake up with new boobs.

The final breasts would be softer, closer together, and more natural looking than my hard-ass expanders, but with the same anti-gravity perk. Like my original set, they would not be perfectly symmetrical, since the left side would always be a little higher and tighter than the right due to the radiation treatment. Still, I was hoping that things would be pointed back in the right direction, if ya know what I mean.

To prep for surgery, I was also eating more pineapple and papaya, which contain natural enzymes like bromelain and papain that can help the body heal faster and reduce scarring. I would also be taking Arnica daily, a homeopathic remedy for healing from trauma, bruising, and injuries. My diet had stayed pretty clean, although I had added in wild-caught fish and eggs for extra protein and the occasional glass of red wine. (Hey, it does have antioxidants!)

Back to the boobie surgery! The recovery was estimated to take five weeks total, with me driving within three to five days and able to lift up to 15 to 20 pounds. I planned to take two weeks off of work and then play the rest of it by ear. Many women had shared with me that the pain wasn't bad at all, that they were off heavy pain meds within a day or so. This was nice to hear, yet I was also well aware that the pain level from the last surgery was WAY more than I expected. Based on that experience, I intelligently set aside the time to heal and just be.

Mom arrived that day, not because her help was necessary for this surgery, but because we wanted to be together for the final chapter of this crazy journey. *I'm so excited!* The night before the surgery, Travis, Mom, and I dined at our favorite Thai restaurant in Uptown, Malai Kitchen, for some vegetarian pho. I'm ready for this pho sho.

It was the day! *New Boobs! New Boobs! AHHHHHHHH! Deep breaths. Inhale. Exhallllllllle....BOOBS!*

The surgery was over before I knew it. My eyes flickered open in the recovery room to see my loved ones surrounding me. Through my foggy, mushy mind, I asked, "Was everything OK? How do they look?" They told me the surgeon filled the implants with 560 cc's. "Wait that sounds big, are they too big?" I looked down. There they were: swollen, weirdly lumpy, and being cradled by the world's ugliest hospital bra. *Dude, these should be illegal.* My plastic surgeon arrived, pulling the curtains closed for privacy. "OK, let's take a look," he said.

I watched his eyes zero in on my breasts—he was concerned, yet extremely calm and laser focused. "OK, the left one is already pulling up. I swear they were even on the operating table. That's just what can happen with radiated tissue. I am going to need you to press down from two different angles 5-6 times per day to help it drop. Try it with me. Press down here. Deep breath in. And out. Repeat." I really appreciated his attention to detail and clear instructions. He was all over this. At the same time, my inner child was whining…more work? *I thought I was done! Ugh.*

Apparently my body did not want to leave this hospital. It would not pee. *Again.* I paced up and down the room, drank loads of water, coffee, anything to try to stimulate my bladder. I found myself in the bathroom singing to myself, rocking forward and backward. I could hear the nurses on the other side of the door:

"Has she gone yet? Seriously?" I picked up a magazine to distract my mind, and right when I was learning the proper way to cut an avocado, I heard the magical trickle of pee hitting the water. After five Goddamn extra hours, I was finally released to go home.

I needed a lot of rest over the next few weeks while the swelling and bruising subsided. My body cycled through a rainbow of colors, at this point leaning towards shades of red, purple, and yellow.

Also, I was very sore. Oddly enough, the area in my hips where the liposuction was done was sorer than my breasts. My low back looked like it had been kicked by a horse. I had to wear a compression girdle around my torso, which was kind of a pain and did not mix well with Texas hot-ass weather. However, to my delight, the physical pain itself was very manageable, almost a breeze compared to the last surgery. I guess comparison does serve after all!

Comparison served, that is, until I began to compare my new boobs with my originals. The new boobs and I were not having the "love at first sight" affair I had anticipated. You see, as with any surgery, they looked worse before they would look better, and I was now realizing just how strongly my mind had been holding an expectation of "instant boobie perfection." I wanted to control the healing process and cosmetic outcome. I was pissed, disappointed, insecure, and impatient. And I didn't want to feel any of it!

Leftie was a couple of inches higher, and if you were standing next to me, my left nipple would look straight at you saying, "Hey! I've never seen life from this angle before." Rightie looked pretty good, more natural, at least until I flexed my pec muscle. It then shriveled up into a squashed, inverted raisin, leading me to become self-conscious in certain yoga poses and during sex. If I was on top of Travis when we were making love, my flexed puckered boob hung right in his face. *Ummm…this was not in the brochure.*

Therefore, I adopted a healthy daily practice of obsessively staring them down in the mirror, examining their weirdness from every angle, comparing them to my gift-from-God original breasts, and then crying. A lot.

One morning while sitting next to Travis on the living room couch, I noticed he was looking through old photos on the laptop. He came across the sexy nakey photos we took right before treatment began. My heart sank into my chest; I felt a nauseating heaviness consume me. He smiled, telling me, "Look at these! They are hot!" and I violently ordered him to shut it down. I couldn't bear looking at the beautiful body I used to have. It hurt too much.

I want my old body back.

This wasn't the first time this thought appeared during treatment. While doing chemo, there was a moment when I was in the bathtub and caught my reflection in the faucet handle. I saw skin and bones...the image of an anorexic, bald, and sick girl.

It was all hitting me again, and hard. I was grieving. It was time to go in. *Is it true that I want my old body back?* YES!!! *Can I absolutely know that that's what I want?* NO. My "no" came from this consideration. What was I more interested in: living a life where my joy was dependent on how my body looked and felt, OR living a life of joy regardless of what was happening with my body? I'll take Option 2, please. *Shit. Looks like I'm really getting my practice.*

When I believed that *I want my old body back,* I felt an intense heaviness in my heart. It wanted to scream, and I wanted it to shut up. It was a vicious, internal war, with me living in constant comparison. Instead of seeing the joy I felt when taking the nude photos, I experienced them as a huge punch in the gut. When I looked in the mirror, all I could see were scars and deformity. I tried to tell myself that they were only breasts— *there's no more cancer, you stupid idiot, you should be happy with what you have.* I became snippy with Travis and wanted to pull away from everyone.

Who would I be without the thought that I want my old body back? Without the thought, it felt like dark sunglasses were removed, revealing the miraculous healing that was taking place in my body. I observed the 16 inches of new scars that painted my torso, and I saw in that map my personal journey of transformation, resilience, and strength. Whoa—the scars even *looked* totally different. I was actually proud of them and what I had been through. *Can I love my body just as it is?* Yes, I could love it in all its glorious weirdness. *Do I need to despise my body in order to take action?* No. I could do my part from a place of peace—ask the plastic surgeon questions, go back to physical therapy, do my home practice, buy flattering bras and lingerie, be gentle with myself, and commit to my inner work. I could also hold myself through the grief.

The photos, when I was ready to look at them, also looked completely different without the thought. I could remember how much fun we had taking these beautiful pictures that captured a special moment in our lives. And yet, these photos weren't *me.* They were just images of the past. When I freed myself from comparison, I was able to admire them without admonishing myself.

I don't want my old body back. Well, this turnaround was actually truer—that old body had some rockin' cancer. I was also remembering how much neck tension and headaches the weight of my natural breasts caused. *Besides, what if this boob situation is my gateway to self-love? Unconditional joy? Would I take a pair of weirdo boobs in exchange for inner peace? Yes. Bring it.* I was learning a new way to compassionately be with myself that could only serve me in the future, especially if I had the privilege of experiencing an aging body. *Gosh, I'd love to get old.*

I want my thinking about my old body back. Oh yes, wow—I wanted to see my body how I used to experience it. I wanted the sexy confidence, the pride of showing it off, the gratitude I felt. However, this was a *mindset,* not a body type. And it was still possible to get that intimate relationship with my body back now.

My body wants me back could also be true. Maybe it wanted me to come back to reality. To see how much it was healing. To pet it, massage it, and love it no matter what. To tell it that it was doing a great job and that I was here for it. It felt good to see my body as my friend, a companion, instead of an enemy.

This inquiry went on over time, of course. I didn't come to these realizations in one sitting. Examples arose out of thin air, while in the shower or on a walk. It was a slow unraveling. While it was unfolding, waves of overwhelming emotions of depression, rage, hopelessness, and loneliness continued to hit me.

I tried to be patient, but my mind was fucking relentless. *I don't get it. I'm DONE with cancer and cancer treatment, why is this happening now? The cancer is GONE. What's going on here?*

Back when I was in the middle of chemo, I attended a cancer support group. With my bald head and tiny body, I shared that I was surprised at how well I was doing—I felt pretty darn good compared to the stories I had heard, and my attitude remained clear and positive. Then the ladies said, "Oh…you just wait until after treatment. You're going to feel horrible." *Oh yay! Fun! Thanks for the heads up!* Then I went on to hear about how terrible their lives are, the side effects from treatment, and how they lived in constant fear of a recurrence. As I witnessed their suffering, I could see so clearly that it was in their minds—if they could just let go of these stories, this victimhood, they would have a happy life (insert spiritual arrogance here). Why couldn't they just see this?

Well, now I knew why. When you're in the midst of suffering, you are bombarded with a torrential downpour of stressful thoughts, images, physical exhaustion, and Big Fucking Emotions

(BFE's). These BFE's produce a dark cloud that looms over you, covering your eyes, so that all you can see is crap here and crap there. You are totally blind to reality, stuck in a terrifying mental movie. I wanted to press the magic button to get out of this shit-storm. Where was it?

I dove right into the deep end of BFE's for the next month. *Oh my God, it's so painful. I don't know how much more I can take.* Much to my surprise, the BFE's of depression, fear, anger, resentment, loneliness, and disappointment were not my biggest problem. Do you know what made these moments completely unbearable? It was thoughts like *I should be happy. There's something wrong with me. It will get worse. These feelings will never go away.*

When I believed these thoughts, I was covering my BFE's with painful sticky notes. Like pouring a pitcher of freshly squeezed, salted lemon juice onto a raw, oozing, open wound, it led to mental and emotional exhaustion. I couldn't take it anymore. And it took a physical toll as well.

In addition to feeling disappointed with the cosmetic outcome, my BFE's were fueled by an upper respiratory infection that created an intense, persistent cough. I coughed so much that I threw a rib out of place. With each inhale, it felt like a knife was stabbing me in the side. On top of that, I had some kind of acid reflux thing going on where I coughed too much after a meal and ended up vomiting. *This blows!* Whiny, annoyed, and just wanting to get back to my normal life, I didn't want to do The Work. I didn't feel like doing movement. Screw it all! I just curled up into my bed and cried.

How do I react, what happens when I believe that I should be happy when I'm not? I was even more frustrated, ashamed, disappointed, hardening inside and wanting to close myself off from the world. I saw images of the "Old Bethany" who was peaceful and free. *Where did she go? COME BACK!!!!* She was lost forever. I couldn't see the possibility of a happy future.

Who am I, feeling this way, without these thoughts? I took my time with this question. *Oh.* Big freaking exhale. *Wow.* I really was here for me. I rocked me through tears, I asked others to hold me. I felt the support of the bed. I told myself, "It's OK, you're doing great, and this too will pass." Ahhhhh…more deep breaths. *Maybe these BFE's are a necessary part of healing? What if I welcome them instead?* So I let myself fully feel. I peeled off the sticky notes and even stopped giving them an emotional label of "depression" or "anger." Without my stories, without putting those extra sticky notes on what I was feeling, the whole experience actually felt quite intimate. *Whoa. This is different.*

One night, I experienced what one might call an "emotional exorcism." Seriously, if there had been a hidden camera in my home, I would be locked up right now. I found myself sobbing, hovering over the toilet, and profusely vomiting. My body was uncontrollably shaking. My husband came rushing in. "Are you OK?" Between dry heaves and gurgled vomit, I managed to get the words out: "I. Feel. So. Fucking. Out. Of. Control." There was no choice but to surrender into what was underneath the pain: complete and utter *grief.* Grief for the changes in my body and in my life. Grief for having absolutely no control over any of it.

With my husband's encouragement, I gave myself permission to fully let the grief and helplessness take over and move through me, which lasted for hours. Cold bathroom tile beneath my knees and a firm white ceramic toilet seat for my arms, my body had support. As painful as it was, there was also a sweet tenderness in my husband holding my sausage curls back from my forehead and comforting me. *Look at how he is showing up for me.* It was as if my BFE's were giving him an opportunity to live his amends, to be there for me the way he wished he could have always been while I was in treatment. I got to live out part of my amends too. I was free to be completely unguarded and vulnerable with him. *It's safe to count on him. It feels so soothing to trust him and let go.*

At some point, he helped me crawl back into bed, massaging my head as I drifted off to sleep. The next morning, I was immediately met with more tears, but I didn't fight them. Wet-eyed, I dressed and drove to acupuncture, where I cried through the entire session. I told myself that I was keeping the faucet on for as long as it needs to be on this time. Until the well was dry, until all of the emotions were emptied. This was an act of self-love. *It's excruciatingly beautiful.*

And all of a sudden, for no apparent reason, it ended. I began to feel lighter, calmer, at peace. I fell into my body and breathed. My smile and sense of humor returned. Life surprisingly looked sparkly again. I felt like *myself* again.

For me, the BFE's could not be bypassed. No spiritual self-talk could shut them down. It was essential for me to really, truly feel them. Let them have a life. Let them move through me. Be authentic. I saw it as an opportunity to love *all* parts of me. The sad me, the crazy me, the confused me. Just like my body didn't define me, these emotions didn't either. They were simply different flavors of my personality, and they were just so innocent. *Wow, I'm really learning how to make friends with big emotions. How to stop fighting them; they have a right to live and be expressed.*

Once I was on "the other side," I did some stream-of-consciousness writing to capture each painful voice, each stressful belief, and take it to inquiry. I wanted to take notes on the inner tape recorder and find out if it was all really true so that I could continue to become enlightened by suffering. *Gosh, suffering is so fucking profound when I completely surrender into it.* Suffering taught me humility, connection, self-care, and the power of the mind.

The timing of BFE's showing up even more after treatment now seemed divinely perfect. I didn't have the distraction of the slew of doctor appointments and had already set aside time for recovery. I just hadn't realized that I was setting that time aside for the recovery of my mind.

In the future, grief would hit me again and again. Thanks to these recent experiences, I now had more proof that it was OK, that I was safe to be with it, and that it was safe to let others, like my husband, in while I was in the shitstorm. The icing on the cake was that this experience trained me to feel safe and available to be with other people's pain too.

BFE's are a natural part of the human experience, including the cancer journey. This time had taught me so much about how resilient I am. I can get through *anything*.

To the women I judged at the cancer support group: I was such an asshole. *I am so sorry.* You are entitled to feel however you feel and process however you want. There is *nothing* wrong with you.

If you are in the midst of cancer treatment, I don't want to paint a scary picture of your future. While PTSD is common after cancer, it is not your destiny. However, it may be comforting to know that if you are feeling it, you are not alone. Please give yourself a huge hug right now and get support. Call a friend, visit your local cancer support center, see a therapist, or call the free Do The Work Helpline found on www.thework.com.

There are many ways to deal with emotions. Venting it out may be the best way for you. For me, it can feel so good in the moment, but it is often not enough. Really feeling my way through it exorcism-style and questioning the beliefs that lie beneath are how I find the most freedom.

I was now free to love my body right here, right now. I continued my practice of daily stretching, massaging, and boob pressing. I was free to laugh about it all too. *I mean, really—this is all just wild isn't it?* And I was *finally* free to fully celebrate the end of treatment and live my life to the fullest.

If you want real control, drop the illusion of control; let life have you. It does anyway.

–BYRON KATIE

16

Out Living It

DID YOU KNOW that if you get cancer, you can go on free vacations? #cancerbonus

I was on my way to a weeklong cancer vacay in Montana. YES, that's a thing! My dear friend Michelle, whom I had met during my adventures in Spain a decade earlier, was joining me. Our friendship quickly jumped to 'Breastie' status when her breast cancer diagnosis arrived six months after mine. How funny it seemed that at one time we were touring Spanish vineyards, sipping Cava, and partying in clubs all night...and then we were texting boob pictures back and forth, asking, "How are your boobs today? Do yours ripple like this? How much hair do you have left?" accompanied by countless words of encouragement.

When she told me about her diagnosis, I had recently learned about these free trips, so we pledged that after we rocked this cancer thing, we would reunite for a celebratory cancer vacay. I couldn't wait to see her.

The event was hosted by First Descents®, an incredible non-profit organization that creates life-changing outdoor adventures for young adults impacted by cancer. The founder, Brad Ludden, nicknamed "Man Salmon," has had a love of the outdoors since he was a small child. He felt especially drawn to whitewater kayaking and must have been pretty badass at it, since at the age of twelve, he was traveling and competing internationally.

At the age of twelve, I was collecting POGs, playing volleyball, and practicing French kissing behind the school's performing arts building.

Both admirable life paths.

Brad's passion became clear when his aunt was diagnosed with breast cancer in her thirties. Witnessing her going through treatment, he noticed how little support there was for young survivors, especially when it came to nature and mental/emotional healing. He began to take her on kayaking trips, which helped to get her mind off of her diagnosis. He then started volunteering at a local pediatric oncology program teaching participants how to kayak. He witnessed the profound effect of the outdoors and adventure and wanted to transform his passion into an act of service. By the time he turned eighteen, First Descents was born.

A first descent is defined as "the first time a person successfully kayaks a river or section of river that has never been done." Brad had traveled all over the world in search of the thrilling challenge of embarking on a first descent.

Brad explained it this way. "I wanted to recreate the experience of a 'first descent' that had so greatly impacted my life for people like my aunt who really needed it. For the last eighteen years we've been humbled by the depths of river canyons, the wonders of summits, and the glow of campfires. In these wild places we are witness to the strength and resilience of our participants who take on rapids, rock walls, and waves and bravely defy their diagnosis.

At FD, cancer is never the defining factor. We don't serve cancer patients. We adventure with amazing young adults in the prime of their lives who are coping with a cancer diagnosis—and that's a critical distinction. Our participants are supportive friends, powerful advocates, and forever our greatest teachers."

I was so inspired by Man Salmon's story. I loved hearing how people create companies and careers out of kindness and compassion—a true business from the heart.

First Descents now leads trips all over the world with adventures ranging from rock climbing in the Cascade Mountains to surfing the California coast to hiking in Italy to whitewater rafting in Costa Rica.

My choice? Whitewater kayaking in Tarkio, Montana.

Stepping off the tiny-as-hell airplane into the adorable-as-hell airport of Missoula (which resembles more of a "rest stop" than an airport), I arrived.

Our camp mom, nicknamed "Butcher," texted me to let me know that there was already a group of participants gathered. "Just look for the big moose head." He would arrive shortly to pick us up and take us to the lodge in Tarkio.

Timid and curious, my eyes scanned the airport searching for a giant moose head overlooking a pile of bald, sick-looking people. Much to my surprise, everyone looked just like me. Healthy and young, with big excited smiles on their faces.

I introduced myself, and the immediate cancer connection took over…the drop-the-BS-we've-been-through-some-major-shit-yet-we're-still-here bond. Within minutes, we opened up about the nitty-gritty details of our diagnosis and treatment plans…boobs were felt, hair compared, photos shared. We talked about our fears and struggles, and the good parts too.

We pulled up to the lodge, which was a massive log cabin tucked away in the mountains overlooking the Tarkio River, and were greeted with ginger turmeric spritzers and vegan welcome appetizers. All of our meals were organic and plant-based—wow! I had attended and hosted a lot of retreats, and this was top notch.

And who was paying for all of this? I learned that numerous companies donate to First Descents, and some of the biggest contributors are pharmaceutical companies. Yes, friends, Big Pharma was paying for my healing, life-changing vacation. Think about that the next time you bash them. I love when the mind thinks it has its labels all figured out—for me, discovering that medicine is a gift has been truly humbling. *Thank you, Big Pharma.*

A new vanload of participants arrived at the lodge, and I heard Michelle's high-pitched voice coming from the front entrance. "Michelle!" We ran towards each other, squealing with joy, nearly knocking ourselves over in a tight, twirly embrace. Happy tears were falling, which sparked the waterworks in some other participants. Flashes of memories filled my mind—Skype videos showing our scars, emergency freak-out phone calls, and celebratory victory dances. I was so grateful for all of it.

A unique FD tradition is the gifting of nicknames. Your old identity is washed away and replaced by something more fun and meaningful. Michelle quickly earned the nickname Diva for the ridiculous quantity of luggage she had brought for a weeklong trip. To her credit, she was also moving from Maryland to Colorado, but I would still have to say the name was a perfect fit.

For two gals who had been in a long-distance cancer friendship and recently had boob jobs, the obvious first activity was to rush down to our room, take off our shirts, and examine each other's boobs. #CancerGirlsGoneWild™

Seeing hers, I was struck with jealousy—they looked amazing! In her type of surgery, the implants were placed over the pec muscles, and they had a very natural look. Because she didn't need radiation for her Stage 1 cancer, she didn't have to deal with the scar tissue and wacky nipple directions like I did.

When I showed her my set, she was very complementary. Then I performed my creepy contortionist boob trick of flexing my pec muscles. Her head flung back in shock, and I burst out laughing. *Ahhhh yes, I'm still getting used to the quirks of this new body.* At least it was now becoming entertaining and hilarious instead of traumatizing. I would later learn the best party trick of all—when I'd stand in a dark room and place a flashlight next to my breast, it lit up like a bright pink glowing ball. Yes, friends—I have #glowboobs and if you have implants—you do too! *Now this is enLIGHTenment.*

My first FD nickname was Terre, short for Cinque Terre, Italy, my favorite place on earth. At dinner later that night, I saw one of the staff members leave to get the last participant at the airport. One who never showed up. Another staff member asked me, "Wait a minute—is your name Bethany?"

"Yes, it is," I replied as I watched the realization sweep over her face that they had sent a staff member to pick me up. And here I was at dinner. We all laughed about how, for a few hours, there were two Bethanys, earning me the new nickname, B2.

The water had a life of its own. In areas, it was as still as a glass stovetop. One small tap from the fin of a fish or the beak of a bird led to endless, swirling ripples that extended to the river's edge. Similar to the ripples in my new breasts, I supposed.

Some areas had strong currents, clearly inviting us to make life easier for ourselves and go with the flow. However, obstacles quickly appeared in our path. Giant rocks and boulders disrupted the flow, creating turbulent whitewater rapids. The adrenaline of adventure kicked in, leaving no choice but to face what lay ahead.

After a rapid, it is common for an eddy to appear to the right or left—a soft, still resting place to reflect on what has just happened. Heartbeats begin to slow. *How do you feel? Did you freeze in fear? Conquer with courage? Did you forget everything you learned and totally bite it? And are you still OK in this moment?*

I was astonished at how at home I felt in the water. When my body slipped into the blue, plastic kayak for the first time, it was natural and familiar. During our training with the Tarkio raft guides—six extremely experienced (and adorable) wilderness dudes—we learned various paddling strokes, what to do when our kayak flipped, and how to ask for a rescue. I was surprised to learn that much of the power and steering did not come from the paddle, but from my hips and shifting of body weight. We were taught the shorter strokes needed to gain speed and how to guide the front tip of our kayak directly into the center of the waves. "Aim for the V! You want to be in the V," exclaimed one of the guides. *Hehehehe, there goes my 13-year-old boy mind again.*

I immediately fell in love with this sport, this art of meditation. I picked it up quickly, my yoga background helping me connect with my body and breath and keep me calm in the rapids and underwater. My body was becoming stronger, more vibrant, and more daring to take risks. My trust in its strength and dependability began to return.

When I was diagnosed, I lost trust in my connection to my body. I had always thought of myself as intuitive and in touch with my inner workings. This was shattered when I had no idea my body had been hosting a cancer party in my left breast and lymph nodes for years. Even when I felt the lumps and watched them grow, I didn't believe it was cancer. Nearly a year passed by before that inner voice kicked in.

I then handed my body over to the doctors, as I saw them as the experts, that they knew what was best. They had the experience with cancer. My body, healing cancer, became their job, and I was happy to place my body in their care. I took care of my body too, but in a way, I thought of it as fragile, delicate. Treatment was very aggressive, so I didn't feel the need to be aggressive with my body. I countered the intensity with a lot of rest and nurturing. My yoga practice became gentler and softer as well.

On the water, post-treatment, and with some new body parts, I could feel my physical power and strength returning. I felt the intuitive force, the trust, and the daring sense of play. *Bring on the fucking rapids.*

It turns out that biting it through a rapid is also hella fun. My body chose to take a spontaneous swim on the biggest rapid of the trip, appropriately named Tumbleweed. "What stage is this rapid?" asked Freckles, a young California girl who had rocked through two rounds of leukemia by the age of twenty-three.

"It's not stages like cancer," I responded, giggling, "It's a Class 3." *Right now, I'm feeling courageous and invincible enough to face anything—even a terminal rapid.*

Before I knew it, I had bounced right out of my kayak after the first big Tumbleweed wave. After gulping down a gallon of ice-cold, metallic-tasting river water, I made my way to the surface, found my paddle, and held onto the side of the boat. I assumed the defensive "swim down a rapid position" with my head up, arms wide, and legs in front of me, so I could bounce my feet off of the rocks instead of smashing my face into them.

It was a strange and surreal feeling being completely at peace in the turbulence. I was actually having fun, perhaps because I had zero clue that the biggest drop of the rapids was quickly approaching. The senior kayaking guide swiftly paddled up the rapid (yes he was a rockstar) to meet me. "B2, what are you doing in the water?"

I responded with a smile. "I'm all good, I'm going to swim this one out."

"NO, you're not! Get back in the boat." He said in a calm, clear, military voice.

Awwww shit. "Are you serious? How?"

His hands grabbed the top of my lifejacket and attempted to pull me up into my kayak, but I lacked the upper body strength to make it all the way in. In amazement, I watched my left leg swing up and over the kayak in a very ungraceful yoga maneuver. I finally hoisted myself back into the boat; he threw me the paddle, straightened my kayak, and a split second later, I flew down the massive Tumbleweed drop.

A huge smile splashed over my face, and I couldn't stop laughing. *What a rush!* I loved it. And I wasn't alone. All of the participants swam parts of the Tumbleweed rapid that day. Furthermore, we all discovered the same truth: what we had feared turned out to be exhilarating and fun.

The river taught us strength, courage, how to go with the flow, and to face what was in front of us, even when scared. Trusting our bodies, nature, and the community of guides and new friends and connecting with others through our struggles and victories made a beautiful metaphor for cancer. And for life.

I left a lot of fear behind in that river. After noticing weird blood stains on the back of my shirt, I apparently had also left a mole behind. It must have rubbed off my back and taken a swim at some point in my kayaking adventure. Perhaps I had wanted to leave a piece of me behind…*remember me always, Tarkio.*

Of all the people I connected with on my FD trip, I learned the most from Zen. She was one of the last participants to arrive. I met her on the lodge's rustic, wooden front porch as she rolled up the ramp in her wheelchair. Struck by her kind, calm eyes, and contagious grin, I reached out for a hello hug. Zen couldn't have been a more appropriate nickname for this beautiful soul.

I immediately wanted to know her story, especially since I had never had a friend in a wheelchair before. At the same time, I didn't want to pry or be rude. *Was she born this way or was it cancer? Does she have any use of her legs? Will the sensation ever come back? What is her life like? How does she feel about it?*

Throughout the week, we had some remarkable conversations, and I got to spend a little extra time with her after the trip in her hometown of Missoula. She was a superhero. I admired her so much. She was also an open book about her experience with cancer and living with what society calls a "disability."

I sat with Zen at a quaint café in downtown Missoula. After ordering coffee and vegetarian breakfast burritos, we started chatting up a storm.

Four years ago, at the age of thirty-one, Zen was a world-traveling, active, young woman living with her boyfriend in Mexico. She had started feeling a little off in her body, but ignored it. When visiting a friend in Portland, her balance became noticeably wobbly. One day, after a hike, her legs collapsed on the flat pavement of the service road. At the persistent insistence of her friend, she finally went to see a doctor. They discovered a large tumor pressing into her lower back. Although it was unclear whether or not the mass was cancerous, it still needed to be surgically removed.

As with all surgeries, there were numerous risks of complications, yet there was only about a 20% chance that she would lose the use of her legs. Being paralyzed for the rest of her life wasn't really on her radar as she prepared for surgery.

After surgery, she opened her eyes to find her surgeon holding her hand. I noticed a tender, heartwarming smile on her face as she recalled how compassionate and intimate it was that her doctor had waited for her to wake up. I could tell that they had formed a special bond, which is often the case with patients and marvelous doctors.

"He was always very protective of me," she said.

She woke up into a new body. A body that couldn't walk on its own, ride a bike, jump in the shower, dance, or travel easily. She woke up into a completely different life. Independence went out the door. Daily life and the simplest tasks became difficult and frustrating.

For her, the first year was really difficult, emotionally and physically. She moved back in with her parents and hated the idea of being dependent on them. One of the great lessons of her journey was to learn how to ask for and accept help from others. I could totally relate. It was humbling.

What helped her the most was continuing talk therapy and physical therapy for two years after her surgery. "Being able to share, cry, and express anything and everything that I was going through was so helpful." She had struggled with depression during different phases of her life, so a low-dose antidepressant had also been very supportive for her mental and emotional well-being.

Throughout the healing process, she maintained a positive

attitude that infected those around her. Even the nurses took notice, telling her that she was the reason they were in this line of work. She also connected with a new community of others who had experienced spinal cord injuries, gaining invaluable friendships, inspiration, and practical knowledge for living in her new body.

Eventually, she realized, "Oh wow, I can do a lot of things! I can push my body. I just have to trust it more."

Over time, she learned how to reconnect with her body and read its cues to know when it was cold or hot, hungry or thirsty, or needed to use the bathroom. One of the coolest things I learned was that she had had a surgery in which the doctors rearranged her body parts so that she was now able to pee out of her belly button. Talk about superhero powers!

"Oh yeah! It's great!" she said with delight. "The other day on the kayak when we were all together, I just went off to the side and peed while sitting in my boat. Super easy!"

We cracked jokes about what a unique talent that was. I loved her vulnerability and openness in answering my questions, and her willingness to share. She was gentle, excited, and engaged.

Four years after her surgery, she had reclaimed her independence, moving out of her parents' house in Oregon and into her own apartment in Missoula with her cat, Raja. She could drive with the help of a special hand gadget for the gas pedal and brake. In addition to her full-time job as a web designer, she was starting her own business. She was a badass on the kayak and also biked and paddle boarded—truly an inspiration to everyone she encountered.

I could see her in a philanthropic role helping others who were newly disabled. Giving TED talks, traveling across countries to share her story. She was the first person I would want to talk to if I found myself with a disability.

Actually, the word "disabled" didn't fit. It wasn't true. She was fully able-ed...pure joy on wheels!

Zen didn't let her diagnosis or paralysis define her. "I haven't let it be an identifying factor. I acknowledge it's part of my life and how I move through the world, but it's not my identity. Getting out there and challenging yourself is important. Some people become ashamed of themselves. Society treats you very differently—like a child, like you can't do things. I used to get angry (and sometimes still do) with others, so now I try to have more compassion. You can be pissed about it or go with it. I choose to be an ambassador and lead by example."

Her eyes twinkled as she described the blessings of this experience. She was happier, had richer friendships, and knew her own resilience and strength, certain she could get through anything.

When I asked her about romance, she told me that she had wanted to find her own stability, her own independent happiness first. I loved that. Now that she was in that space, she was ready to start exploring romance and learning more about how her body responded to it. I chimed in, "Perhaps there's a landmine of unchartered orgasmic spots in your body just waiting to be discovered!"

"Yeah! I'm pretty excited," she said with a curious smile. I tentatively asked, "So would you say that cancer has made your life better?"

"Oh...Absolutely...I am such a better person than I was before cancer."

"And would you trade it? Would you take your old life and your old body back if you had the chance?" I asked.

"No, I wouldn't." she responded.

"Me neither."

We both giggled in amazement as the goosebumps popped up on our arms. A moment of silence to take this in. *Wow.*

It was one thing for me to say that cancer is a blessing… I mean geez, all I did was get some new boobs. Zen was really living it. Words can't describe how much I admire her, and that's why I wanted to share her story with you. Whatever life brings you, whatever challenges, it is here *for* you. All you need is the willingness to see it this way.

Don't be too careful. You could hurt yourself.

BYRON KATIE

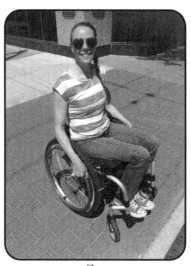

Zen

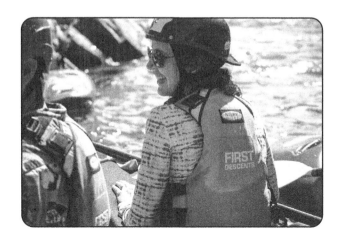

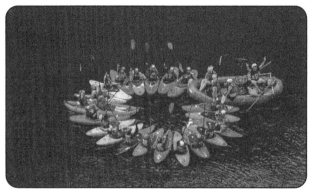

First Descents Family

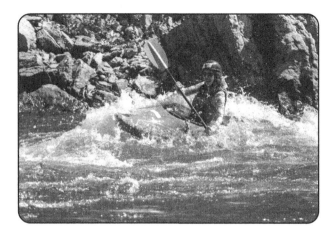

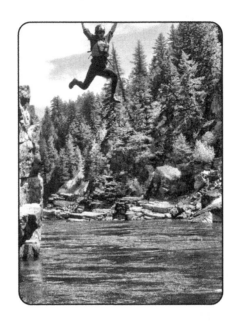

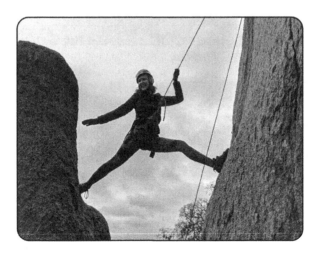

17

Healing in Mexico

IF YOU ARE WONDERING HOW to celebrate the end of the cancer journey and re-ignite a marital spark, I have one word for you, and it rhymes with shooloom.

Tulum. Sweet, sweet Tulum, Mexico.

It was the perfect finale for our two-year adventure and the perfect medicine for healing our hearts. The bridge between a life of treatment, doctors' appointments, and uncertainty to living a full life, enjoying the moment and each other.

We arrived. Eyes wide open, gasping at the ocean view from the balcony of our bungalow, I giddily ran down the bamboo stairs towards the blue clarity of the water. The warm sand filled the spaces between my toes, and the cool breeze tickled my cheeks. I fell back on a plush beach bed for a moment of stillness to take it all in. *Wow, we did it. And we are here. Here, together.*

The first night, we hopped on bicycles and pedaled through

the jungle and down the long, winding dirt road like little children. Riding behind Travis, weaving in and out of traffic, I caught glimpses of his endearing dimples. *He looks so happy and free. And damn, he has nice calves.* I loved how often he peeked behind him to check in on me…most likely to confirm that I had not been run over or kidnapped by a Mexican cartel. He just couldn't shake that masculine protector role.

We pulled up to Hartwood, a chic new restaurant. They were booked up months in advance, but Travis managed to snag us a rez. So much for my story of Travis not being a planner—he had planned this entire trip. And he did it well. It turned out that this was the trip to Mexico he had been saving for, a much better trip than the one he'd originally imagined.

One of my favorite evenings was the salsa night at the neighboring resort, La Zebra. Cuddling on a couch, tucked away from the crowd, we sipped local craft beer and watched the array of salsa talent. The eight-piece band was having the time of their lives, completely in sync with one another. And the dancing! Gorgeous women confidently shaking their hips as they were spun around by their partners and then embraced in a heart-opening backbend. Both athletic and sensual, it left me with one thought: *I need to learn this dance.*

One dancer, who I dubbed Red Dress Lady, caught my eye, a young woman in her late twenties with long blonde wavy hair down to her mid-back. A tight red dress clung to her hips, barely making it over her butt cheeks and exposing her back. She was in her element. I watched her bounce enchantingly from partner to partner, fully enjoying and embracing the moment and movement. *Yup, I want be her when I grow up.*

But someone else grabbed my attention more. A little two-year-old girl with a mop of ringlet curls on top of her head plopped down right in the middle of the dance floor. My heart melted the moment I saw her swaying to the music without a care in the world. Then she pulled her signature move—she clasped her chubby fingers together over her head, tilted her head and arms forward slightly, and proceeded to twirl in circles over and over again until she face planted on the floor. Mom then swooped in for the rescue. The little girl laughed and did it all over again. Twirl. Fall. Repeat.

Why do images like this touch our hearts so much? In this case, I believed it was because I saw myself in her. I saw the small, innocent, carefree child in me who loves to unapologetically dance like nobody's watching. The part of me that can let life spin me out of control until I fall flat on my face. The me who could still manage to find enjoyment in it, even the falling. The me who gets up and is willing to do it all over again.

Red Dress Lady and Twirl Girl inspired us to step away from our comfy couch and onto the dance floor. Without a clue about how to salsa, we were forced to make it all up. Just two kids, moving and grooving our bodies and laughing at ourselves. With every beat, I could feel the heavy seriousness of the past slip off of our shoulders.

Our days were spent doing as little as possible. Sleep in, make love, walk the beach, swim, lounge on the beach bed, eat, drink, nap, repeat. We did attempt to be "productive" and "adventurous" one day and tour the Tulum Mayan ruins, but the heat and the crowds quickly sent us right back to our favorite beach bed.

For my part, I tried to blend in with the locals by wearing as little clothing as possible. I had bought a yellow string bikini to house my new boobs, which had me feeling pretty damn fabulous, even if my pale and pasty skin might have blinded some of the tourists. *This. Girl. Is. On FIRE!*

Quite literally on fire. By Day 3, I was a lobster, looking like I had taken a long soak in a bathtub of beet juice. Ya know, the exact opposite thing you're supposed to do after having gone through radiation. *Oops!* Responsibly, I started sitting in the shade under an umbrella, wearing copious amounts of sunscreen, draping a towel over my legs, wearing a long-sleeve shirt, and donning a hat. But still sexy, of course.

During our last sunset, I grabbed Travis's hand and dragged him into the ocean with me to go body surfing. A storm had recently blown through, leaving unusually big waves for the Tulum coast. We hopped over each one, screaming at each other. "Whoa— did you see that one?" When a ride-worthy wave approached, we yelled, "This one! This one! Let's do this one!" This went on for hours.

I loved the feeling when you catch the wave at that perfect moment, right when it's about to topple over you. There's the thrill of the initial drop, and then I'd shift my body into the locust pose position with my arms extended forward, core and legs engaged, balanced by a softness in surrendering to the water around me. The current and bubbles thrust me forward towards the coast until I felt the rough sand beneath my belly, inviting me to come up for air. I felt like a mermaid dancing through the waves.

When I was little, *The Little Mermaid* was my all-time favorite movie. I wanted to be Ariel. Perhaps that's why I became a redhead in my early twenties? My childhood girlfriend, Sterling, and I would play in the pool for hours reenacting the scene where Ariel throws herself onto a rock with the waves crashing behind her as she belts out the climax of the song, "I wish I could be…part of that wooooorld!!!" One of us would be Ariel (OK, I probably hogged that role), and the other would splash the water into the air behind her. It was SO realistic.

After I was diagnosed, Sterling mailed me a gift that contained a kids' puzzle of *The Little Mermaid*. Her mom was also a breast cancer survivor and had been so loving and supportive. They would even soon offer up their home in Colorado to help me finish writing this book. I love the moments when you feel like every single person you know is so meant to be in your life.

Travis and I continued swimming, surfing, and laughing in the water until the tips of our fingers looked like raisins. It felt timeless. When we needed a rest, we floated further away from the shore, past the break of the waves. My legs wrapped around his waist as we kissed until a wave filled our mouths with saltwater.

For our last dinner, we restaurant hopped, ending the night at our favorite vegan restaurant, The Real Coconut. Eating chocolate cake and sipping Argentinean red wine, we curled up together on a soft white loveseat under the stars. We felt like "us" again. *Ahhhh, what a relief.*

The rediscovery of this slow, simple, carefree, and adventurous aspect of our relationship was exactly what we needed to hit the reset button as we returned to our new life in Dallas. The trip didn't actually heal our marriage; instead, it reminded us of the passionately strong connection that still existed between us. It was a connection that was never lost, merely buried under a shitload of stressful thoughts and BFE's. We now had the motivation to continue to work through our challenges. It has taken a lot of time and patience. And it hasn't always been easy. We've been calling it our "relationship rehab" phase.

Although it appeared to have been a delayed reaction (but what do I know about the timing of life?), the cancer experience did strengthen our relationship. I am now free to be totally honest with him. We have the rawest conversations. We talk about the possibility of divorce—where we would live, how we would split up possessions, how we would continue to help raise Nainoa. We talk about what we find attractive in other people and ask ourselves how we can bring those elements into our marriage. We share what we appreciate about each other and what doesn't work for us. We get clearer on where we'd like to see our lives go from here, the desire to be more spontaneous and free, like we were when we first met. There is nothing I can't say to him now. It's truly liberating.

Will we be together forever? I honestly don't know. I can picture a beautiful life without him too. And the idea of being on my own and counting on myself is really attractive. But I can't know the future and after all, I could be dead soon. Regardless of what happens, I do know we are free to stay or go, live or die, with love.

We are love and there's nothing we can do about that. Love is our nature. It's what we are without our stories.

—BYRON KATIE

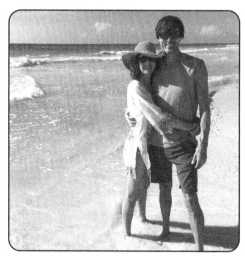

Beach Babes

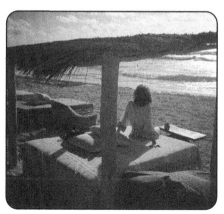

Beach Beds

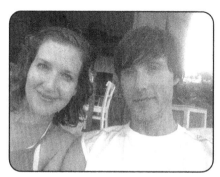

Tulum Shooloom

18

~~Dying~~ *Living from Cancer*

ONE NIGHT, I had a vivid dream that I was dying. I was lying propped up in a hospital bed inside a roller skating rink (totally normal, right?). Along the outside of the rink stood all of my family and friends, everyone who has ever touched my life. In front of an audience, the doctor told me that the cancer had spread to my rib cage and spine and that there was nothing more they could do. The cancer was terminal. I was to make my final preparations and say my farewells.

I thought to myself, *I'm dying? Whoa…this is it.*

A complete acceptance and peace washed over me. I was then being slowly pushed around the rink to say goodbye. I saw smiling faces, tears, my hands touching theirs, connection. Then I noticed my breath start to shorten and my body feeling weak. *OMG, this …is….what…dying feels like.*

Then the realization hit me, *Wait a minute…right before*

receiving the news, I was actually feeling pretty great and now my breath just disappears and my body shuts down? I was all good until I believed I was dying. Could this just be in my head?

Suddenly, a surge of resilience arose. *I'm not dying. Right now, I am actually alive...but only in reality! I'm alive until I'm not. I'm going to make the fucking best of the time I have left.*

My hospital bed and I were wheeled out of the rink towards a new room. Through the opening of the sliding glass doors, I spotted a computer from the 1980s: old-school, boxy, and grey.

I heard the words: WRITE.

Suddenly, I snapped out of the dream and woke up in my bed, startled. *Where am I? What just happened?* I quickly looked over and saw Travis sleeping. *Oh my god, it wasn't real. It was all a dream.*

But damn, I got it! Message received. I'd been procrastinating turning my blog into a book, and it was time to return to my writing. It didn't even feel like a choice, more like something I knew I had to do for myself. Time to birth my book baby into the world.

So here I am, many months later, sitting on the porch overlooking the serene mountains of Vail, Colorado, where I am living this season because life is way too short to spend summer in Texas, and I'm writing the last chapter.

I am truly grateful and blessed to be someone who can say the words, "I used to have cancer." My latest CT scan showed no evidence of disease. *Cancer-free, baby! Cancer is over. Or...is it?*

The truth is, cancer has already come back many times...in my mind (and apparently in my dreams). The fear of cancer returning and doing so terminally offers a big opportunity for me to practice.

Yes, I'm aware it's all mental, but holy crap—that fear can take me for quite a ride! It's like a vampire who sucks the joy out of everything. It's the voice that says, "Don't get too excited…What if…?"

The fear is also ignited by ANY new physical sensation I feel in my body. If I have a cough, *It's in my lungs!* If my low back hurts, *The cancer has spread to my sacrum!* Recently, there was even a throb in my toe…so obviously, *There's a tumor in my toe!* This can get pretty exhausting, as well as pretty entertaining at times.

I now work with many cancer survivors who are afraid to be happy. One client talks about how she will find herself doing something she enjoys, like shopping for a new dress, when "reality hits." The reality that cancer could come back at any moment. Her pleasure switches to anxiety, fear, and panic.

I invited her to stay in this experience to see what was *really* going on. *What is "reality" in that moment?* The reality was that she was happily living her life, shopping for a dress. And then, boom… the "What-ifs" marched in carrying scary images of the future. Was this real or an image? Did "reality" actually hit? Or did she get whacked by imagination?

Imagination hit. Our mind thinks that we should proceed with caution. *Don't get too excited, suffering could be just around the corner.* In other words, our mind thinks that we should suffer now to prevent future suffering, as if a constant state of worrying can actually prevent disease. It's totally insane!

And if the fear of cancer returning isn't enough in life after cancer, guilt also rears its ugly head. *You should just be happy there's no cancer, other people are dying and suffering, you asshole!* This voice has a label: Survivor's Guilt. While I have experienced it many times myself, it's also really fascinating to explore the logic behind this way of thinking: since other people are suffering, I should suffer too. Since other people are dying of cancer, it's somehow rude and inconsiderate—even arrogant—to be happily living my life. Therefore, I should be in misery, or at least politely hide my happy dance. This will obviously make them feel good and make the world a better place.

Can you absolutely know it's true? Does it actually work? Not in my experience. Katie often says, "What I love about separate bodies is that when you hurt, I don't."

But when I believe you are deeply suffering, I project my imagined experience onto you. I am imagining what I would feel like if I were dying of cancer, and then I scare the shit out of myself. I am reacting to my own imagination. Can I really know that's *your* experience?

When I am not consumed by thoughts of you suffering (which is really me suffering in my own mental movie), I become available. I am fully present for you and for me. It's 100% compassion. I can be happy, live my life fully AND be connected with you. It's an "and," not an "either/or." I can ask you with an open heart, "How you are doing with all this? I'm here for you. How can I help?"

I know that if I were on my deathbed, which could happen at any time, the last thing I would want is for others to withhold their happiness in the name of "my" suffering. Talk about dying with a guilt trip! I would much rather leave this world knowing that others are fully embracing their lives. To everyone reading these words, if you hear I'm about to die or I'm already a corpse, you have my permission to enjoy the fuck out of your life. In fact, if you don't, I'll butterfly stalk you and whisper "Is it true?" into your ear at night until you wake up to your beautiful life.

I haven't always had this sense of humor and acceptance around death; it's been slowly cultivated through inquiry. Just like I've been a student of cancer, I've become a student of death. This practice started back at the retreat in Quebec with Tom Compton. Tom was amazing, one of those connected, special souls who was put on this earth to inspire others to live a fearless, joyful life, simply by being himself. Life had given him many surprises as well; his wife had recently passed away from breast cancer.

Hearing him speak of his time with his wife as she transitioned inspired me, showing me how death can be an intimate, heart-opening experience for a family. I also loved seeing how well he was doing. He had moved to California and started surfing every day. Tom exuded a child-like charm and had somehow figured out how to reverse the process of aging—he looked twenty years younger than the last time I had seen him. *He used to be grey, frail, and walking with a cane. Now he's blonde, buff, and surfing?*

At first, what I had feared most about death was how it would affect my loved ones, especially my husband. Travis has already had to deal with so much loss and death; it didn't seem fair for him to lose me too. I shared this with Tom, who told me, "It would break his heart. And then it would break it wide open."

While I found comfort in his words, I also started to ask a lot of questions. "How did your wife know the cancer had returned?" She was in alternative treatment, so I knew there weren't a lot of diagnostic scans.

As soon as the words left my mouth, my mind spoke up. *EEK! Are you sure you want to know this? The answer is totally going to screw with you.*

And I still wanted to know.

He said that her stomach became very bloated and they found tumors all along the lining of it. From that point, it was only a matter of time. I felt an immediate pain in my stomach. However, I kept a brave face and moved to the next conversation topic.

So of course, naturally, for the first half of the retreat, my stomach became bloated. It was crampy. I started obsessively feeling it for lumps. *Oh crap, this is it.*

One of my main intentions for joining the retreat was to confront any remaining fear and unease around my diagnosis. I could see that this was the perfect time for me to experience these sensations. It was happening *for* me. Throughout the retreat, I did a lot of inquiry into my fear of death, fear of having chosen the wrong treatment plan, and fears of my family suffering.

There was a lot of crying. It felt tender and kind to let the little terrified girl inside of me fully speak, and I also felt very held and supported by Tom and the other retreat participants. It became clear that a bloated belly was not a problem—it was what I was believing about it that hurt. Cancer returning was not a problem. Even death wasn't a problem. It was the labels I put on them that created my suffering in those moments. It was that dang scary mental movie…again! I heard Katie's words, "It's our thoughts about death that scare us to death."

Then one afternoon, I quietly snuck up to the retreat home's attic, which had been converted into a large, rustic A-frame bedroom with a private bath. I filled the porcelain claw-foot tub with warm water, sprinkled in essential oils of frankincense and lemon, and slowly slid into my thermal, comforting cocoon. I looked down at my bloated-as-hell belly and caressed it. *Hey, you.* Wiggling my legs straight, I began to lean into a delicious forward fold. And something astounding happened.

I farted for about 30 seconds straight. It was the longest wind relief I've ever experienced. I burst into laughter—farts are always entertaining to me, as I grew up with brothers and we have so many fond family fart memories. *Did you know you can save one in a jar and give it to someone as a gift? Oh wait you didn't? You're welcome.*

When I sat up from my forward fold in the bath, my stomach was flat and back to normal. My giggles turned into an over-whelmingly grateful big ol' ugly cry. My fears. My terror. All along, it was just a fart. The next day, my menstrual cycle made an appearance after a six-month hiatus.

This got me thinking. How often have I experienced fear and it turned out to be absolutely nothing? Or maybe my fear came true, but it turned out to be a blessing in disguise? What if fear is simply an entertaining, farty friend, inviting me to get out of my head, let go (pun intended), and enjoy reality?

All flatulence aside, The Work really does show me HOW to make peace with my nightmares, and the ultimate nightmare is death. So I have been going deeper in my exploration of death.

In fact, death has become a welcomed, fascinating meditation. You're dying. I'm dying. We're all dying. As Katie says, "Let's face it, bodies don't make it." No medication, supplement, prayer, meditation, exercise, or amount of money will prevent you from transitioning out of this body.

So why do we spend so much time fearing it? Why is death considered a worst-case scenario? A bad thing? What beliefs am I holding about death and dying that make me terrified of it, that prevent me from looking forward to it?

Here's what comes up for me: *Death is painful. Death is bad. Death means failure. My loved ones will suffer. I can't live a full life while dying. I will die with regrets. I can prevent my death. I will miss out.*

And WHERE did these beliefs come from? *Where's my proof?* I realized that my personal stories of death mainly come from movies. Literally, Hollywood has taught me death is painful, horrible, and something to be avoided. On film, it's not only painful for the person dying, everyone around them suffers too.

My second source was stories from other people about how tragic death is, although none of them have actually experienced death themselves. So my version of death is a combination of

Hollywood and second-hand stories. *Hmmm…..this sounds like solid evidence that death sucks. Could each of my death beliefs be total BS?*

Of course, I take my deadly thoughts to inquiry and find my own truth. The truth is that I absolutely cannot know that any of it is true. I've never died before.

How do I react, what happens when I believe these deadly thoughts? I am 100% incapable of enjoying my life in the present moment. The grim reaper lurks over everything, over any new physical sensations, scan time and doctors' appointments, taking walks, cuddling in bed, going to work, driving my car. It's suffocating.

Who would I be without these thoughts? The side effect is so strange. I'm actually getting excited about death. I'm actually curious and looking forward to it! *What will it be like? I wonder when and how it will happen?* Ohhh wait…a pain in my gut, a tug in my heart says, "BE CAREFUL! If you make peace with death, you will die even sooner! That's how you create your reality! You were excited about cancer, and then look what happened!?"

Oh, sweet, innocent superstitious mind. *Can I absolutely know that this is true?* I can create the timeline of my life? I can control when I die? Where in the world is my proof of that? It's just another trick of the mind.

How about the turnaround? If I make peace with death, I will not die sooner. I will die perfectly on time, in peace. So far, the only things that are really dying are my beliefs. Inquiry is killing them off, one by one.

I know what you're thinking (OK, wait, I can't know what you're thinking…more accurately is that I know what I think you're thinking)—it's easy for me to be at peace about death since I don't have a terminal diagnosis. It's all just theoretical right now.

You're totally right. I can never know for sure what my reaction would be. But if I can make peace with cancer, I can make peace with death too. This is my new favorite question to contemplate...*How would I live if I knew I was dying?*

That time between my diagnosis and waiting to find out how much the cancer had spread was two of the most incredible weeks of my life. All of the daily bullshit stressors completely dropped away, and I found myself in an astonishing state of gratitude for everything and everyone. I experienced joy in the simplest of pleasures, like riding the trolley, watching Nainoa's soccer games, cooking a meal, sitting under a hot shower, holding hands with my husband, even stepping on acorn shells (not kidding—there is something SO gratifying about the crunch of an acorn!).

As I try on this scary future and let myself feel through the terror, I see an opportunity for even more presence, slowing down, and deeply connecting with my loved ones. Appreciating every second that I am able to be with them.

I see sharing my experience of dying with others and learning from others. I see acceptance, peace, and gratitude for every moment that I've been given. I see forgiveness—making amends with others and within myself for anything that still hurts.

I see traveling more when/if it's an option for my body. If I can't travel, I see asking my friends from all over the world to send me short thirty-second videos of the inspiring places they go and things they do so that I can experience the world through their eyes, from my hospital bed. I see writing letters to my loved ones, letters they can open after my passing as a way for me to continue to be with them.

I also see opportunities to totally screw with them...making random requests in my will like "all family members must wear a chicken suit to my funeral." Cremation actually sounds really cool, and they now make biodegradable urns that you can plant into the earth...then a giant Bethany Tree will bloom on top. *Wait a minute…can my Foobs be cremated? Or will I be left with a pile of ashes and two great boobs? Seems like they should at least be recycled…*

Back to my death meditation…*how would I live if I knew I was dying?* I'd say YES to life more often…I'd try that salsa class, jump on a surfboard, go whitewater kayaking, float in a hot-air balloon. I might even move my life to a new place, one surrounded by nature, adventure, and community.

I'd continue to take care of my mind with self-inquiry and would question thoughts like *I am dying…can I absolutely know it's true? Or is it truer that in reality, I am still here breathing? Is it possible that I am even more alive than I have ever been?*

I'd love on my body, giving it nourishing foods, movement, time in nature. I'd love the shit out of that piece of chocolate cake and glass of wine too.

Any part of aging would be a celebration. Finding a grey hair or wrinkle? *Yes, please!* Grey hairs would mean I've had the privilege of growing older.

To be clear, I'm not saying it would be easy. I'm very confident I'd have some pretty stellar freakouts, and just like I did throughout this cancer journey, I'd get to learn over and over again that I'm still OK in each moment. I can feel the intimacy of being with myself in that deep pain and suffering, as well as the intimacy of surrendering my entire body weight into someone else's arms.

Being at peace with death doesn't mean I won't seek out the best treatment, do what I can to heal my body, or feel frustrated, lost, and hopeless sometimes. When I fall apart, inquiry is always here to hold me, to bring me back to the kindness of reality. Death may be the kindest offering from the universe. The ultimate coming home. A way out of pain. I can't tell you how comforting this awareness is.

So…WHY wait? I can live ALL of this now. Perhaps the

turnaround to my question is truer: *How would I live if I knew I was ~~dying~~ living?*

With an open mind, death is a catalyst for truly living. This contemplation on dying is giving me the perfect prescription for how to fully embrace life *now*. Not in 5 or 10 years, because that time isn't guaranteed for anyone, *so how about now?* In this moment, I can honestly say: I am open and willing to die, if that's what reality brings. And someday, reality will bring it!

Speaking to people with more direct experience with death has also supported me in dropping my fears; now I have a handful of "good" death stories imprinted in my brain, and that list is growing.

My dear friend and client, Nancy, told me about her mother who was advised by doctors that she had two months left after her bladder cancer had metastasized. She walked straight out of the office and said to her daughter, "Do you know what my diagnosis is? Live every day to the fullest." Now that's a clear direction. Two years later, she passed in peace. And passed her enlightened thinking onto Nancy.

Shortly after her mother's death, Nancy's husband passed away from terminal liver cancer. After working through the grief, she transformed her entire life. She retired to Florida, where she teaches Zumba, feels healthier than ever, and has met a wonderful new man. She says, "This is honestly the happiest I have ever been. Why did it take me so long to figure all of this out?"

A client from New Zealand shared with me that her uncle was diagnosed with terminal cancer. When he was ready for in-home hospice care, all of their close friends and family literally moved into the home with him. Together they cooked great food, sang songs, told stories, and celebrated life. He died within two weeks. My client said it was so much fun, so inspiring, that nobody wanted to leave.

I know people who have technically died, they say they've flat lined, and each one describes death the same exact way: as being overcome with the most comforting, all-encompassing, indescribable *peace*. Have you read Anita Moorjani's *Dying to be Me* book? Her experience of death was breathtakingly beautiful, yet she consciously chose to come back and share the message for us all to live a fearless life by being ourselves. I am reminded of Byron Katie's words, "Death is so sweet, few people come back to tell us about it."

Remember my courageous yogini friend, Lonne, who was diagnosed right before me? The one who inspired me to get my lumps investigated further and to openly share my journey with others? She transitioned out of her body within five months. Hearing the news of her death, especially while just beginning my own cancer journey, shook me to the core. Yet later, spending time with her partner, Todd, and learning about all of the incredible ways he still feels her presence and connection transformed my fear into curiosity and wonder. *Is death even real?*

Her passing left him without a home, and as the universe would have it, our old B&B retreat property, Living Waters, needed a new on-site manager. Obviously, we recommended him for the job. He's been happily living there and growing the business for over two years now. Life is fascinating, isn't it? It's all for me. Even cancer, even death. It's all a gift.

A few months before I jumped into this epic summer in Colorado to finish my book, I visited my childhood home in Ft. Myers, Florida. A two-story ocean-blue wooden house with white trimmed plantation shutters. My parents were selling the house, and I tried using my cancer card to prolong the inevitable clean-my-child-hood-shit-out task for as long as possible. *It's time.* I climbed up the carpeted staircase, the same staircase that as young children, we would patiently wait at the top of on Christmas mornings, bouncing up and down, until we got the parental thumbs up to race down and see Santa's prezzies. I strolled by the white wooden door to my parents' room that used to house my two long strands of curly hair—perhaps that was not an attractive touch for the showings.

At the end of the hallway, I opened the door to my old bedroom-turned-guest room. I smiled at the love seat next to the windowsill where I would journal, draw, and stare out at the blue sky and green palm trees. Plopped down on the carpet in front of my ginormous mess of a closet, I dove into old photos, clothes, home schooling projects, artwork, and hand-written notes from friends. A piece of paper stopped me in my tracks. It was a feed-back form I had filled out describing my experience after our 9th grade Outward Bound trip in the Florida Everglades. When asked what I learned from spending a showerless week canoeing with my classmates in a smelly, alligator-infested, mosquito-filled swamp, I wrote, "I have learned that the only way to get through tough times is with a positive attitude. The worst of times can turn into the best of memories." *Whoa. Wait a minute. This is exactly what I've learned, 20 years later, from cancer.*

Was this wisdom within me all along?

Did *cancer* actually teach me? I mean, did the cancer cells jump out of my body, develop mouths and voices, rub their Buddha bellies, and impart upon me this knowledge? Or, in reality, was my greatest teacher…*me?* Maybe a curveball like cancer was needed to coax this awareness out of me. More proof that life's shit really is our fertilizer for self-growth.

By shifting my perception to see life, death, cancer, pain, doctors, medicine, my husband, child, parents—*all* of it—as teachers, I was able to open the door to this knowingness within me. I needed to point the finger "out there" and use inquiry to find my truth in here. *What if we all already have the magical juju we need to move through any challenge life brings? What if the rumors are true: we are our own Gurus?*

Sitting next to my husband at a Byron Katie event in Los Angeles, my heart begins to race. In front of an audience of 400 or 500 people, I confidently raise my hand, grab the mic, and stand up. I inhale deeply, look into Katie's crystal blue eyes with gratitude, and begin to share how much The Work has shifted my experience of cancer—my experience of life. After I finish, she asks, "Which would you rather have…a body that is free from cancer or a mind that is free from cancer?"

Before I even have a moment to consider her question, I hear the answer leap out of my mouth, "A free mind."

Freedom from cancer is a state of mind.

—BETHANY WEBB

TOP 10 LESSONS FROM MY GURU CANCER (ME)

1. Cancer is never a problem. It's what I'm believing about cancer that hurts.

2. Cancer shows me how to live in and embrace the present moment.

3. Cancer invites me to see kindness and support in everything and everyone.

4. Cancer helps me to slow down, listen to my body, and see it as a friend.

5. Cancer teaches me self-love, acceptance, and limitless strength.

6. Cancer opens my heart and helps me live a richer life rooted in gratitude.

7. Cancer shows me how to make friends with medicine, seeing it as God too.

8. Cancer inspires me to follow my dreams now and live a fearless life.

9. Cancer teaches me how to make peace with and surrender to the unknown.

10. Cancer opens my mind to find the gifts (and humor) in everything life brings.

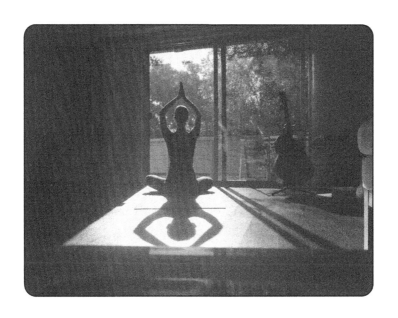

EPILOGUE

A Born-Again Breastie

September 4th, 2020

Today rings in my 39th birthday, nearly five years since my "new direction day" diagnosis, and I'm holding this precious book baby in my hands. Yep, I'm still alive, my friends! And one might argue I'm more alive than I've ever been.

Even though there isn't proof of one single cancer cell left in my body, I still use it as a guide for how to live the fullest life possible. It's like I have a #livelifenow fire under my ass fueling me. And it's led to some very big decisions, most of them beautiful along with one utterly heartbreaking one.

A little over a year ago, I found myself behind the wheel of my white Toyota Camry hybrid, jam-packed to the brim with everything I owned (which apparently was not a lot). The mountains were calling, and I was leaving Texas, my home for 20 years, for a fresh start in Colorado. With *Frozen's* "Let It Go" blaring on the speakers and expansive flatlands and windmills in my rearview mirror, I slid my wedding ring off my finger —this move, this transition, was for me.

Choosing to shift my relationship status from married to friendship was one of the hardest, most gut-wrenching decisions I have ever made. I wish following my heart didn't have to break someone else's.

A month after our return from Tulum, Travis and I had faced another crazy life challenge, and the same dynamics revealed themselves. Me, trying to make the best of it, doing what I could to improve the situation, and letting go where I had no control. Travis, living in fear, emotionally checking out, and not fully showing up in our marriage. It became clear to me that this partnership wasn't working for me anymore.

After coming home from a rock climbing trip and a solo retreat at Living Waters, I sat Travis down on our L-shaped couch in the living room. Yes, that same couch where we held each other in tears hearing those three life-changing "you have cancer" words. I told him that I couldn't do this anymore and wanted a trial separation. I needed to experience life on my own. I needed to rely on only me. To put my desires first. To follow my adventurous, independent, nomadic spirit that I had discovered during my time in Spain. His initial reaction —a mélange of shock, anger, and hurt —is forever etched into my heart. The separation was set for the summer, four months from then.

Following our tradition of being nontraditional, we chose to spend those four months living together in Dallas and making the best of the time we had left. Honestly, a lot of that time was empowering and beautiful —a sweet way to honor our love. It was also ridiculously hard at times. We went into therapy, read about *Conscious Uncoupling*, and did The Work with a Certified Facilitator. We both wanted this transition and decision to take place with as much love as possible. We even wrote an agreement we titled "Time Apart and Within" outlining our guidelines for the separation, including how often we would speak, if we could date other people (not an awkward conversation at all!), and our commitment to staying open, honest, and loving. Dorky me may have even created a logo for it. We agreed to set aside six months.

But I knew within six weeks. I was undeniably so much happier. And after what I've been through, I deserve to not just live—but to feel fully alive. And it's *my job* to do so. It was time to trust that inner voice again. To love myself completely and give myself all of the things I had been craving in my marriage. We are now divorced and are working on our friendship —it has been much harder than I anticipated. I think that old cliché is true: time will heal. I have so much gratitude for my life with Travis, and as sad as I am that the marriage has come to an end, it's also the start of a beautiful new beginning.

I have never been so wildly in love with where I live —every day in Colorado is a new adventure. Summer and fall are filled with hiking, climbing, and exploring, while winter and spring send me to the slopes where I'm pretending to be a speedy ski bunny. For the first time in 20 years, I get to live near family and even had the honor of being here for the birth of my baby brother's first baby, Josephine. Thanks to First Descents, I walked into a loving, supportive community of new friends, and I now volunteer and organize monthly events for them. My career continues to focus on helping others find freedom, peace, and self-love through life's curveballs, especially in chronic health challenges.

My body is doing pretty dang awesome; my energy is back, yet I still seem to be the slowest hiker in every group. These Coloradans are in some serious shape! This teaches me patience and an ongoing practice of *Who would I be without comparison?* to support me, especially on the side of a mountain when a 90-year-old man sprints by me while I'm gasping for air.

I rock my follow-up appointments every six months, and I'm just so beyond grateful to have the extra eyes and expertise on my body. My new tradition of #flowersforfollowups where I hand out yellow roses to the patients and staff in the waiting and infusion rooms brings so much joy to my heart —if you feel any anxiety around doctor appointments, this is the perfect way to brighten someone's day while distracting your fearful mind. Do it!

And how are my boobs, you ask? Well, we just celebrated our three-year boobieversary. Leftie has finally settled down a bit and still flaunts quite the lazy eye. Righty has relaxed so much that I think she can do flips, and she often resembles a dangling plastic bag. Oh, but can they rock a tank top! Yes, I do still get self-conscious sometimes. A revision surgery may be in my future but for now I'm enjoying staying out of hospitals and in nature instead.

As excited as I was to start dating again for the first time in twelve years, I was also terrified. Having had cancer, new weird body parts, and being divorced before the age of 40 didn't exactly feel like the best romantic résumé. *Ummm, when do you mention these things? Will I scare them away? Wait—if someone bolts after I share my story, wouldn't that actually be a good litmus test? Like, thanks for showing me who not to be with*! I know cancer can come back any time, and I want to be with a partner who can enjoy it with me. I questioned beliefs like *cancer makes me a less attractive partner, my boobs will scare men away*, and *I'll never find love again.* With the support of inquiry —OK, and a few glasses of wine —I mustered the courage to fill out my first online dating profile with schoolgirl giddiness. *EEK*!

Just like my thoughts about cancer, it turns out my beliefs about re-entering the dating scene were total BS. I've had the time of my life dating half of Denver lol; I wasn't looking for anything serious and felt free as a bird. Would you like to know the secret to dating?

Being completely at home with yourself, staying present, and having zero attachment to the outcome. I met some amazing men —and a few sketchy ones too —and also spent plenty of time and space with myself. It's all a practice of learning and growing, isn't it?

And then on a snowy Tuesday evening, I had dinner at the Dushanbe Teahouse with a Boulder boy named Tim. Tall, dark, handsome, funny, adorable, intelligent, adventurous, easygoing, not-in-my-plans-but-yes-please, Tim. We hit it off immediately. And suddenly all my desires for dating lots of dudes melted away.

A month later, life gifted us a global pandemic! But I'm not kidding folks —cancer has 100% trained me for COVID-19. It's like the whole world got a cancer diagnosis together since we're learning to live in the unknown, embrace the present moment, slow down, cherish what truly matters, surrender control, have some serious freakouts, and take care of ourselves and each other.

Of course there are some days when I just want to dart out the door without thinking about germs, hand sanitizers, and masks. Run wild in the streets and hug a bunch of strangers. Or at least my Texas/Florida family. Geesh, especially my now high schooler Godson, Nainoa, who I don't get to see as often anymore. That part is painful. And do I also long for the day I can jump on a plane for a spontaneous getaway? *Heck yeah*. But is it true that I want these things right now in the height of a global pandemic? *Actually, no*. It's so clear to me that fighting this reality is utterly pointless. So instead, I'll follow the simple instructions of stay mostly at home, wear a mask, hang six feet apart, wash those hands, and make the best of it.

I've been #coronacoupling with Tim for over six months. It's turned out to be the perfect recipe for falling in love and appreciating the preciousness of life all over again. And cooking. And eating. A lot of eating. I know in my heart that I am all I need, and I'm also so excited to see where this adventure-ship leads.

This new life and perspective wouldn't be possible if it weren't for My Guru Cancer. Every single day is still truly a gift, whether or not I choose to see it. (And sometimes I just can't and that's OK too.) As I sit in my quarantined bungalow in Boulder reflecting back on the past five years, I'm in serious awe of it all. What a crazy. Beautiful. Weird. World.

From the bottom of my heart, *thank you*. Thank you for hearing my story and being with me on this journey. It is my hope that everyone finds true freedom from cancer. A freedom that exists with or without cancer cells living in the body. Thanks to this beautiful practice of inquiry, I'm not a victim of cancer. I'm simply an eternally grateful student, curious and ready for the next Life Guru to appear (whoever or whatever it may be!).

9 months later...May 27, 2021

That's weird. Why is the doctor calling already? I had a low back MRI only two hours ago.

"Hello, this is Bethany."

"Hi Bethany, this is Dr. I. Are you sitting down?"

Their diagnosis: Stage IV Metastatic Breast Cancer.
My diagnosis: Live the fuck out of life!

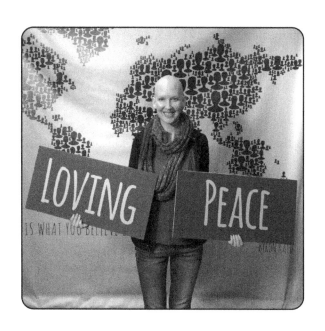

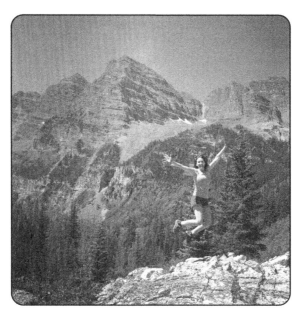

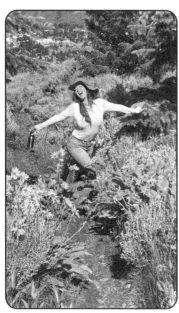

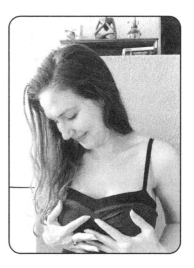

APPENDIX

Resources for Finding Your Own Freedom

NOW IT'S YOUR TURN. Here's my invitation: Look at the challenges you are facing in life, whether it be cancer, a global pandemic, disability, miscarriage, death of a loved one, divorce, addiction, job loss…how could it be possible that this is *the best* thing for you? What is it teaching you?

I'm not trying to negate the fact that there are tough times and struggles…this BFE Earth School can feel REALLY frustrating! I'm inviting you to notice *what else* may *also* be going on…open your mind to the gifts that are all around us. In every moment. Perhaps you already have the greatest guru at your feet, just waiting to be discovered. Invite it in and wake yourself up to this beautiful thang called reality.

How do you wake yourself up? Inquiry. As you've seen in this book, The Work of Byron Katie is a simple yet profound process of identifying and questioning thoughts that create stress and suffering. It's a way to stretch, open, and unwind the mind to fall in love with reality, just as it is.

The Work consists of four simple questions and some turn-arounds. Anyone with an open mind can do it, free of charge, anytime, anywhere. When you are feeling stressed, the invitation is to pause and notice what you are thinking and believing, then write it down and investigate its validity using The Work. The four questions are:

1. *Is it true?*

2. *Can you absolutely know it's true?*

3. *How do you react, what happens when you believe that thought?*

4. *Who would you be without the thought?*

The turnarounds are a way to experience the original stressful thought from different perspectives, by looking at opposites. They open the mind to seeing other possibilities in life, possibilities we are blind to when we are under the influence of a stressful thought.

There is definitely no shortage of stressful thoughts in the cancer experience! Cancer can touch every aspect of our lives: health, body, relationships, finances, career, family, creativity, spirituality, and the fear of death. Cancer has given me the ultimate invitation to live this practice. Here is a sampling of my own stressful thoughts from The School of Cancer:

Painful thoughts about cancer: *I have cancer. The cancer is spreading. I want it to go away. Cancer is a life-threatening disease. Cancer makes my life more difficult. Cancer prevents me from living a full life. The cancer will come back.*

Fears about treatment: *I don't know what to do. I will make the wrong decision. Chemo is poisonous to my body. Medicine isn't spiritual. Treatment is painful. The pain will get worse and never go away. I am nauseous. I can't handle it. I will deal with a lifetime of side effects.*

Judgments about doctors/medical system: *Western medicine doesn't treat the whole person. I want the doctor to tell me I don't have cancer. The medical system/insurance/labs should be easier and more organized. The doctor didn't prepare me for this. I want the surgeon to be kind to me. I need doctors to heal me.*

Self-blame/judgment: *I created my cancer. I could have prevented it. I should have lived a healthier lifestyle. I should be able to heal myself on my own. I shouldn't feel this way. I need to know the test results. I need to be strong. I'm doing it wrong.*

Body image: *My body betrayed me. My body is too skinny, sick, and unattractive. I am no longer feminine. I want my old body back. My body is unhealthy and full of toxins. I am losing my breasts. That little boy should know I'm a girl.*

Relationships: *My husband doesn't agree with my treatment plan. I am a burden to others. My partner is not attracted to me. My mom should stop worrying about me. People shouldn't pity me. My clients will not want to work with me. People look down on me because of my treatment choices.*

Fear about money: *Cancer is expensive. We need more money. Cancer will financially ruin us. I can't afford these medical bills.*

God: *God should cure my cancer. I need God to explain to me how and why I have cancer. God is cruel. God is punishing me.*

Fear of death: *Cancer will kill me. I will die young. Death is painful. Death means failure. People around me will suffer. If I die, it's my fault.*

Sound familiar? You might relate to many of these thoughts even if you don't have cancer. Ya know why? We all have the same BS (belief systems) floating around in our minds. We are connected in this way. And we can break free from the pain by exploring our mental dis-ease: our thoughts. Where are you frustrated? Where are you arguing with reality? What I love about The Work is that your pain is your gateway to freedom.

Everything you need to know to start your own practice of The Work is available, for free, at www.thework.com. You will find helpful videos, worksheets, a free helpline, events, books, audio recordings, and more.

For additional mental and emotional support for the cancer journey, check out www.CanSurround.com, for inspiring and informative articles, thought inquiry (The Work of Byron Katie), meditation, yoga (led by me!), sound healing, online journaling, and more. If you're ready to turn cancer into a true adventure and connect with other young thrivers, visit www.FirstDescents.org.

To work with me via coaching, online programs, or speaking events, head over to www.mygurucancer.com. Follow my journey @mygurucancer and subscribe to my email list for the latest news, inspiration, freebies, silly musings, and more. It would be my privilege to connect with you.

ACKNOWLEDGMENTS

SO MANY HUMANS HAVE INSPIRED ME in my journey of cancer and the birth of this book baby. First and foremost, I want to thank my beautiful, compassionate, rockstar of a mother —Debbie Padnuk. You were with me for every step even though you lived miles away. I could not have maintained this level of sanity without you. I'm so grateful for you. To Travis, I love you. Despite the challenges, you have been my lover, best friend, held me through my tears, and encouraged me to follow my dreams —especially my writing. You are always in my heart. To Nainoa —you constantly show me how to keep life playful and see the silver linings. Thank you for letting me into your life and becoming family. Thank you to Angel Elaine for your support and connecting me to the right doctors when I needed it most. To all of my amazing family members in Florida and Colorado: Dad (Drew Padnuk), Ryan Padnuk, Annie Padnuk, Jordan Padnuk, Emma Trucks, Arya Padnuk, Leela Padnuk, Josephine Padnuk, Rocco Padnuk. Thank you for your unwavering love, caretaking visits, and for making this life even more beautiful. To Tim Adair for showing me that love is always possible and for constantly cheering me on, especially during the book baby birthing process.

Big hugs to Byron Katie and Stephen Mitchell for developing a practice that has forever changed my life. Thank you for your continued commitment to end suffering in the world. To The Work community and countless facilitator friends who supported me: Roxann Burroughs, Robyn Povich, Meg Maley, Tom Compton, Susan Vielguth, Sarah-Maya Côte Jirik, Jodi Patsiner, Helena Montelius, Corrina Gordon-Barnes, Todd Smith, Karen Zackowicz, Stan Kurtz, Wendy Davidson, Manfred Friedrich, Edie Thomajan, Tamami Fujiwara, and the many helpline volunteers. You held my tender heart so compassionately as my mind opened through inquiry. This book would not exist without you.

This journey would have been a total shitshow without the love and support of some amazing friends: Carah Ronan, Hadley Palmer, Sherin Barte, Kara Fogelsong, Krissy Kolesa, Sol O'Donnell, Lauren Buck, Alma Fuentes, Jessica O'Keefe —thank you for answering my panicked phone calls and keeping me positive. To the gems Katherine Baronet and Tori Webb Pendergrass for blowing me away with kindness by throwing me a fundraiser. And to those who donated their talents to the event and supported me financially through GoFundMe: you all brought me so much peace of mind during my financial freakout and showed me the generosity of human nature.

To my editor, Jo Eckler, for giving me the confidence that this book deserves to be heard and for your expertise in making it better. To my team at My Word Publishing —Rich and Victoria Wolf —for your guidance, patience, momentum, and oh-so-stunning brilliant book cover design. You have brought this book to life.

To my Texas and Colorado medical teams…you have completely transformed my view of Western medicine. You are such a gift in this world. So much gratitude to Dr. Al for the incredible acupuncture and Kenny Kolter for the gong baths, Reiki, and sound healing. For all of my amazing nurses…you have no idea the joy you bring to the lives of your patients with just a simple smile (and that happy juice doesn't hurt either).

To everyone I've met who is also on the cancer journey —especially the First Descents community and the readers of my blog. A special shout out to Tara Coyote, Michele "Leadfoot" Friedmann, Amy Shields, Mackenzie Squires, Michelle "Diva" Bernstein, Leah "Zen" Zins, Jamie "Mistle Toe" Shadid, Shanna Nasche, Kathleen Groppe, Crystal "Blue Dot" Owens, Cody "Click" Sowa, Maritza "Mañana" Figy, Lisa McMahon, Carlo Lopez @thecancerpatient, and my beloved girlfriend who is making heaven more beautiful: Lonne Dickerson. We are bonded for life and I admire your strength and resilience. To all the breasties who touched my boobs right when we first met or let me touch theirs…it's weird but I'm into it.

Thank you to my Facebook family who kept rooting me on in dark and light times. You literally filled my cup with inspiration to continue writing and sharing. Big love to friends like Nancy Litzler and Christy and Doug Speirn-Smith who gifted me beautiful homes where I could finish writing this book baby (hopefully your couches aren't stained with my tears). To my yoga clients who stuck with me throughout treatment and let me start yoga classes by making them rub my bald head for good luck, especially Shelby Dabney, Heather Molthan, Hillary Dormer, and the Park Towers Ladies. You rock!

To every single student who has joined me for coaching, an online series, or a group training: You are what keeps me going with this work. Hearing feedback like "I'm having a love affair with my illness" and witnessing your ability to free yourself from the most stressful, frustrating life circumstances blows me away. What a fucking privilege. Your commitment to your inner work gives me the fuel to keep going in mine.

I'm sure I have forgotten some names —I'll blame chemo brain (yes, I'm still exercising the cancer card). Please know if we've crossed paths, you have touched my heart, and I'm incredibly grateful.

And last but not least, a big thank you to the lulus that brought me to where I am today: My Guru Cancer.

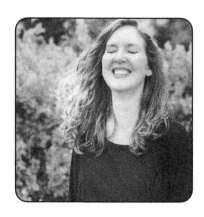

ABOUT THE AUTHOR

As a Mindset Coach, Yoga Therapist, and Cancer Thriver, Bethany Webb's mission is to find freedom with everything life brings. Working in the health and wellness industry for over a decade, she is fascinated by the relationship between the mind and body—how our BS (belief systems) affects our emotions, physical sensations, and overall wellbeing.

Her background provided the perfect training and inner support system to meet cancer with an open mind and enjoy the ride. Late-night writing sprees and a burning desire to share her newfound freedom led Bethany to chronicle her journey on her blog and social media in hopes of helping others transform their own health challenges. Cancer may have rendered her body infertile with two new weird AF boobs, yet it didn't stop her from birthing her first book baby into the world: *My Guru Cancer*.

More than ever, Bethany is inspired to share her story and these healing tools through social media, coaching, online trainings, and speaking events. She now resides in Colorado where you can find her hiking, skiing, adventuring, cooking, loving, and living life to the fullest.

CONNECT WITH BETHANY

www.mygurucancer.com

Follow her journey
@mygurucancer

Sept

Made in United States
North Haven, CT
17 February 2023

32765890R00154